the
NEW
Fat
Flush
Foods

Also by Ann Louise Gittleman, PhD, CNS

The New Complete Fat Flush Program

The New Fat Flush Cookbook

The New Fat Flush Foods

The New Fat Flush Journal and Shopping Guide

The New Fat Flush Fitness Plan

The New Fat Flush Plan

Fat Flush for Life

Zapped

The Gut Flush Plan

The Fast Track Detox Diet

Hot Times

Ann Louise Gittleman's Guide to the 40/30/30 Phenomenon

Eat Fat, Lose Weight Cookbook

The Living Beauty Detox Program

Why Am I Always So Tired?

Super Nutrition for Men

How to Stay Young and Healthy in a Toxic World

Eat Fat, Lose Weight

Overcoming Parasites

Super Nutrition for Menopause

Beyond Probiotics

The 40/30/30 Phenomenon

Before the Change

Your Body Knows Best

Get the Salt Out

Get the Sugar Out

Guess What Came to Dinner? Parasites and Your Health

Super Nutrition for Women

Beyond Pritikin

Eat Fat, Lose Weight for Kindle

the *NEW* Fat Flush Foods

ANN LOUISE GITTLEMAN,
PhD, C.N.S.

Mc
Graw
Hill
Education

New York Chicago San Francisco Athens
London Madrid Mexico City Milan New Delhi
Singapore Sydney Toronto

1 2 3 4 5 6 7 8 9   LCR   22 21 20 19 18 17

ISBN   978-1-260-01206-4
MHID   1-260-01206-9

e-ISBN   978-1-260-01207-1
e-MHID   1-260-01207-7

This book is dedicated to the memory of
my beloved parents Edith and Arthur Gittleman
who nourished me in every way!

Contents

Acknowledgments

My heartfelt thanks are extended to Fat Flushers throughout the world who have embraced my program so wholeheartedly and achieved such astounding weight loss and healing results. I especially want to acknowledge Linda Leekley, who was so very instrumental in the creation of the first edition of this book.

For this new edition, I must personally acknowledge how helpful and wonderful Valerie Burke was to work with. Kudos to her for her expertise and scientific assistance with this project. Also, my most sincere thanks to my staff on the home front. To Stuart Gittleman for facilitating and managing all the "moving parts" with ease and professionalism—as always. To Ally Mortensen, my brand manager, for her critical eye and capable administrative ability. To my editor Cheryl Ringer for always being there no matter when and where. Thanks also to the rest of the dynamic team at McGraw-Hill Education, including Christopher Brown, Donya Dickerson, Ann Pryor, and Chelsea Van Der Gaag.

My continuing appreciation goes out to First for Women, including Bauer Publishing Company CEO Hubert Boehle, Bauer Media Sales President and Publisher Ian Scott, Editor in Chief Carol Brooks, Deputy Editor in Chief Maggie Jaqua, and their exceptional staff who are always a joy: Melissa Gotthardt, Melissa Sorrells, Rebecca Haynes, Lisa Maxbauer, Julie Relevant, Brenda Kearns, and Jennifer Joseph. Beth Weissman from *Women's World Magazine* has been another wonderful supporter who is a pleasure to work with. Also, to my tireless agent Coleen O'Shea who has picked up the mantle from the one and only Nancy Hancock—my first editor.

Introduction

The right Fat Flush superfoods can sweep toxins out of your system to restore optimum weight and well-being better than any "magic bullet" on the planet. *The New Fat Flush Foods* will empower you to finally drop that stubborn fat, reenergize your system, banish bloating and food cravings, tamp down inflammation, boost cardiovascular health, enhance immunity, reduce joint discomfort, diminish digestive issues, and clear your skin while helping to erase wrinkles and age spots—once and for all. But knowing exactly which of the most healing superfoods are the very best for your first line of daily defense is key, and that's where my *New Fat Flush Foods* truly shines.

It is more important than *ever* before to use food as medicine, because today we live in an increasingly toxic world. Each and every one of us is being challenged by a virtual tsunami of health-disrupting environmental toxins, electropollutants, artificial hormones, and chemicals. The sobering statistics published by the nonprofit Environmental Working Group back in 2005 say it all: over 280 toxins and chemicals were found in newborn babies from all over the country. There were 94 chemicals that were identified as brain and nerve toxins, 79 characterized as causing birth defects, and 76 connected to brain and nervous system toxicity. No wonder obesity and degenerative, inflammatory, and autoimmune disorders are skyrocketing like never before and are nearly epidemic. I don't know anybody who hasn't been touched by the illness or death of a loved one due to cancer—an occurrence almost unheard of back in the day when I was growing up.

I dare say that clean, organic, and non-GMO foods are way beyond just a path to successful weight loss. In this day and age, the food, spices, and supplements you choose can be absolutely life-changing. They can also make the difference between life and death.

But let's put the environmental assaults aside. Simply consider the overwhelming and conflicting information about diet these days. No wonder everyone is confused about what to eat. Is it Paleo, primal, ketogenic, vegan, or raw foods? It becomes more confusing than ever to choose your body's preferred eating plan tailored to your unique biochemistry. And that's where *The New Fat Flush Foods* comes into play. Not just a companion guide for the *New Fat Flush Plan, Cookbook,* and *Journal and Shopping Guide,* this book is a stand-alone that will help build vitality and strength with the invincible immune system you deserve while flushing away fat with "superfoods" that are timeless and science based—Mother Nature's miracle workers.

Nutritionally dense, a Fat Flush superfood stands head and shoulders above the most common fruits, vegetable, fats, proteins, beverages, and seasonings you'll find popularized in the "hottest" diet trends or in other bestselling health books. Fat Flush is different from any other eating plan because it features healing gems that flush fat from the body, detoxify the system, and contribute to overall health and beauty. And that's just for starters. Because a cleansing diet is the most important factor in losing weight and maintaining overall health, I've chosen the best of the best— 70 Fat Flush foods, spices, and supplements that contribute to a fit, younger-looking body while you revitalize and rejuvenate your system.

Using the very latest research combined with ancient wellness wisdom, I've put together all you need to know about the premier foods known to burn fat, boost your metabolism, detoxify your body, protect against toxins, and tamp down inflammation while maintaining optimum cholesterol and blood sugar levels. In fact, I've categorized each of the 70 items so that you can know at a glance how they contribute to weight loss. Throughout this book, the following basic categories, or factors, will guide you on your Fat Flush journey toward better health and fitness:

- *Blood-Sugar Stabilizer*
  Foods with this designation are known for steadying your blood sugar, which serves to curb your appetite and prevent the fatty deposits that are part of "insulin resistance."

- *Cholesterol Zapper*
  Foods that help rid the body of cholesterol or help balance the ratio between "good" and "bad" cholesterol levels are identified by this two-word description.

- *Detoxifier*
  To earn this designation, foods must be known for ridding the body of toxins, thereby creating a cleansed and invigorated liver, which is

ready to function as a fat-burning machine and filter for environmental overload.

- **Diuretic**
  Foods that help drain the tissues and eliminate excess water weight (often a sign of inflammation) are in this category.

- **Energizer**
  To carry this designation, a food must fight fatigue, ward off stress, and provide an energizing boost to the entire body.

- **Thermogenic**
  These are foods that raise body temperature, thereby helping the body to burn fat efficiently rather than storing it as fuel.

I encourage you to become familiar with each of the 70 items detailed in this book. By highlighting your shopping list with these Fat Flush superfoods, you'll say goodbye to weight gain, bloating, and those stubborn fat deposits on your hips, thighs, and buttocks while repairing and detoxifying your entire body. However, this book is just one of the pieces of the Fat Flush puzzle. In addition, I invite you to explore the complete New Fat Flush Plan, which details even further how to use these fat-flushing foods to increase your metabolism, eliminate bloat, and speed up fat loss as you reenergize and reset your hormones.

The New Fat Flush Plan goes beyond the conventional answers by uncovering the root causes of why we gain weight and get sick. It is an exciting breakthrough program, already in use by millions of people who are discovering both short-term weight loss and long-term wellness and relief from autoimmune illness.

Fat Flush redefines detox. For over 25 years, Fat Flushers have shown that the program is way more than just a physical cleanse. Their whole life takes on new meaning, and many break through barriers they hadn't had the clarity to navigate before. Whether it is quitting an old job, leaving a "toxic" personal relationship, or pursuing a new hobby that nourishes their soul, men and women of all ages and stages of life have found Fat Flush an elevating life journey enabling them to have a fresh perspective on life and move forward.

Yet even with just this book by your side, you can begin your own personal reset and renewal process. You can also eat your way to weight loss, beauty, and overall good health. By learning about these 70 Fat Flush foods, spices, and supplements, you'll be informed and in control of gaining the fit, tight, healthy body you've always wanted.

1 Fat Flush Staples

The biggest room in the world is the room for improvement.
—ANONYMOUS

My breakthrough detox diet, the New Fat Flush Plan, contains key elements—designated here as Fat Flush staples—that trigger cleansing as well as fat and weight loss safely and simply. Fat Flushers everywhere are discovering this new paradigm shift in weight loss and lasting weight control: the liver—with the help of free-flowing and decongested bile—is the primary fat-burning organ in the body, and it must be cleansed and supported in order to achieve peak performance.

Your liver is strongly affected by a poor diet. In fact, a liver overloaded with pollutants and toxins is the number one weight loss roadblock. Excess fat, sugar (especially fructose), alcohol, and caffeine—along with antidepressants, over-the-counter drugs, prescription meds, and birth control pills—work to sabotage your weight loss efforts by creating a tired and toxic liver and clogged-up bile that can't efficiently burn body fat nor eliminate toxic waste. The New Fat Flush Plan is designed to clean out the liver, promote healthy bile, and help you drop a size or two in up to two weeks!

This groundbreaking diet doesn't stop at flushing fat, as you have read in the Introduction. Fat Flushers have also found that it improves circulation, increases energy, balances hormones, stabilizes mood swings, induces sound sleep, improves skin texture, makes nails stronger, and helps to lessen depression and anxiety. They also report lower cholesterol (as much as 30 points) and balanced triglyceride levels as well as normalized liver enzymes in blood tests. In addition, the added bonus of internal cleansing provides unexpected mental and emotional benefits. A clean body translates into clearer thinking and mental alertness and creates the impetus for change on all levels—whether it is finally cleaning out your 10-year-old files, or straightening up your desk, or getting a brand-new wardrobe.

The Fat Flush staples detailed in this chapter—like coconut oil, avocados, chia, flax seeds, and apple cider vinegar—are crucial to the success enjoyed by many Fat Flushers around the globe. From the initial three-day tune-up and two-week detoxification phase to the second phase of metabolic reset to the third phase of lifestyle eating, the New Fat Flush Plan depends on each of the following superfoods to perform its individual magic. And by working together, these Fat Flush staples transform your body by rejuvenating the liver and accelerating fat loss from your body's favorite fat storage areas—your belly, hips, thighs, and buttocks.

APPLE CIDER VINEGAR

Fat Flush Factors

Cholesterol Zapper
Detoxifier
Energizer
Thermogenic

An excellent fat burner, apple cider vinegar (ACV) helps whittle away excess weight and revs up the metabolism. In fact, a recent Arizona State University study found that participants who consumed as little as 1½ tablespoons of apple cider vinegar ate 200 fewer calories at the following meal. That's amazing, considering that ACV is nothing more than freshly pressed apple juice that has fermented at room temperature for a few weeks.

The main ingredient in apple cider vinegar, acetic acid, is a powerful nutrient that has been proved to stimulate the metabolism. ACV also contains dozens of other nutrients that work to eliminate fat by creating the ideal chemical balance in the body. Researchers at the University of Sydney found that consuming vinegar with meals can lower blood sugar by as much as 30 percent. The acidity in ACV helps slow stomach emptying, which means that food takes longer to reach your small intestine and bloodstream. As a result, carbohydrates are digested more slowly, thereby lowering blood sugar levels and keeping the appetite in check.

Apple cider vinegar contains potassium, which helps transfer nutrients to your cells and give toxic waste substances the boot. The beta-carotene found in ACV also helps cleanse the body by getting rid of free radicals, those unstable molecules that can damage fat, protein, and even our DNA. In a spoonful of cider vinegar, you'll also find pectin, a fiber that "scrapes" the cholesterol off blood vessel walls. ACV is also full of enzymes and amino acids that assist in the development of healthy protein in the body. Studies in Japan have demonstrated that ACV reduces cholesterol and slows down the aging process by destroying free radicals in the body.

Could there possibly be more? You bet. Apple cider vinegar helps cleanse and tone the digestive tract, increases circulation, soothes achy joints and sore muscles, and gives skin a healthy sheen. Pick up a bottle of apple cider vinegar today, and you'll be on your way to a lighter and lovelier you!

Recommended Usage

Up to two teaspoons per day, mixed with water, in recipes, or as a salad dressing.

Just the Facts

- In 400 BC, Hippocrates, the father of medicine, recognized the powerful cleansing, healing, and germ-fighting qualities of apple cider vinegar.
- Apple cider vinegar makes a terrific pH-balancing bath and adds shine when used as a hair rinse.

Boost the Benefits

- When shopping for cider vinegar, look for brands that are certified organic, unfiltered, and unpasteurized. Read the label carefully because some companies sell apple cider "flavored" vinegar.
- Apple cider vinegar requires no additives or preservatives. And there's no need to worry about bacteria such as *E. coli* affecting ACV (the way it might affect apple juice) since *E. coli* can't survive in vinegar's acidic environment.
- Apple cider vinegar should be a rich brownish color with visible sediment. The cobweb-like strands floating in a bottle of natural ACV are edible protein substances that are referred to as the "mother." Having a mother in your bottle of cider vinegar is a *good* thing because it indicates that the vinegar is all natural.
- Organic ACV has a pleasant, but pungent, odor and taste, sometimes causing you to pucker up.
- Store your apple cider vinegar in a dark cupboard to protect the vital nutrients.

Fat Flush in Action

- Make a thirst-quenching drink by mixing a teaspoon of apple cider vinegar with a tall glass of water.
- Before cooking, soak fish in apple cider vinegar and water for a tender, sweeter taste.
- To create a fluffy meringue, beat three egg whites with a teaspoon of ACV.
- To tenderize meat, marinate it overnight in apple cider vinegar and your favorite herbs and spices.

IT'S BEEN SAID . . .

Apple cider vinegar and flax oil make a terrific salad dressing. I use it every day and have lost 25 pounds in three months.

ELAINE T., TEXAS

AVOCADOS AND AVOCADO OIL

Fat Flush Factors

Blood Sugar Stabilizer
Cholesterol Zapper

Avocado is a unique fruit from the laurel family boasting a bounty of healthy fats, fiber, flavor, phytonutrients, and fat-flushing power. Avocados are also known as "alligator pears" because of their pear shape and bumpy skin.

The fruit owes its rich, creamy texture to the high fat content—it's simply loaded with monounsaturated fats proved to lower inflammation, protect your cells from damage, and trim off body fat, especially troublesome belly fat. Science shows that people who consume avocados are much healthier than those who don't.

Fat composition varies tremendously by variety, ranging from 40 to 80 percent. About 80 percent of the avocado's fat is monounsaturated, in the form of oleic acid. Its profile also includes omega-9 fats, the most satiating type with known benefits for appetite, glucose, and insulin levels. Monounsaturated fats in avocados and avocado oil dramatically increase antioxidant absorption—up to 400 percent. Not only are the avocado's own antioxidants more bioavailable, but adding diced avocado or avocado oil to your food ramps up the nutritional benefit of the entire meal. Monounsaturated fats also raise your body's production of adiponectin. What is adiponectin? It's the most significant fat-burning hormone that you've probably never heard of. A 2014 study found that rats given avocado extract showed significantly increased production of adiponectin. Working in tandem with leptin, adiponectin is produced by your adipose tissue and boosts your metabolism by increasing the rate at which your body breaks down fat. Higher adiponectin means better metabolism.

Avocados and avocado oil offer great protection for your heart, including blood pressure stabilization. Avocados are the richest fruit source of phytosterols, a special group of fats with anti-inflammatory benefits for your cardiovascular system. Numerous clinical studies extol the value of avocados for heart health. Avocados' fiber and chlorophyll content support liver function and detoxification. Chlorophyll (responsible for their green color) binds to toxic heavy-metal ions so they can be more easily flushed out of your body. The fatty alcohols also suppress inflammation in your skin, protecting it from UV-induced cell damage.

Other phytonutrients in this amazing fruit include lutein, zeaxanthin, alpha-carotene, and beta-carotene. Avocados' unique nutritional profile helps the body to more easily convert beta-carotene into the active form of vitamin A. These phytonutrients are invaluable members of your cancer-prevention arsenal.

Avocados provide 35 percent of the daily requirements for vitamin K1, 30 percent of the folate, and 20 percent of the pantothenic acid (vitamin B5). They are a source of many other essential vitamins and minerals including vitamins C and E, B6, niacin, riboflavin, and magnesium. An avocado contains more potassium than a banana!

Avocado oil is pressed from the pulp, as opposed to the seed, and has about the same polyphenol content as kale—but tastes better! One study found that eating avocado oil led to better overall liver function, reflected by improved albumin, bilirubin, glucose, and triglyceride levels. The oil also decreases gum inflammation, reducing periodontal disease–related bone erosion, and also helps heal wounds and skin problems such as psoriasis.

Recommended Usage

Eating half an avocado per day is a great way to boost your fat-flushing efforts.

Just the Facts

- The Aztecs considered avocados a fertility fruit, and the Mayans used them as an aphrodisiac. Avocados appear in early Aztec drawings, suggesting South Americans have been enjoying them for up to 10,000 years.
- California grows 90 percent of the American avocado crop with nearly 5,000 growers. Hass is the most common variety, accounting for 95 percent of the supply.

Boost the Benefits

- A ripe avocado will yield to very gentle pressure, without feeling squishy. If the avocado has a slight neck, rather than being rounded on top, it may have ripened a bit more on the tree and have a richer flavor.
- Avocados should not be refrigerated until they are ripe. Once ripe, they can be kept refrigerated for up to a week.
- The area of the avocado highest in nutrients is the flesh nearest the peel, so be careful to not cut away the outermost dark-green portion of the flesh when peeling it.

- Avocado oil is best used within six months of opening. Look for organic, extra virgin, unrefined, cold pressed.

Fat Flush in Action

- For easy pit removal, using a knife, cut the avocado in half by running the knife around its long perimeter down to the seed. Then using both hands, gently twist off the top half. With the pit-containing half in your nondominant hand, grasp a sharp knife in your dominant hand and carefully give the seed a firm tap with the sharp edge of the blade, so that it sticks. Then simply twist the knife—and voilá! The seed magically pops out. With a little practice you'll be a pro.
- Avocado oil has a relatively high smoke point, at least 400 degrees Fahrenheit.
- Although avocados are typically eaten raw, they are delicious warm as well.

Be a Fat Flush Cook

- Guacamole—of course!
- Add to smoothies or blend a few slices into fresh vegetable juice for increased creaminess, satiety, and nutrient absorption.
- Blend avocado into salad dressings.
- Try avocado in ice cream or pie recipes or in increasingly trendy avocado chocolate pudding.
- Brazilians regularly add avocados to ice cream. Filipinos make a dessert beverage by pureeing them with sugar and milk.
- Try an "eggvocado"—an egg baked into the center of an avocado half.
- Drizzle avocado oil over fruit.
- Use avocado oil on the grill for brushing on meat, veggies, fish, or poultry.
- Avocado oil makes terrific mayonnaise.

Fat Flush Fun

- Avocado oil has one of the highest skin penetration rates, so is excellent as a moisturizer. Because of its anti-inflammatory, antiaging, hydrating, and regenerative properties, the oil is effective for repairing cracked heels or dry cuticles and as a moisturizing hair treatment.
- A little avocado oil on a cotton ball is good for removing makeup.

BONE BROTH

Fat Flush Factors
Blood Sugar Stabilizer
Cholesterol Zapper
Detoxifier
Energizer

Bone broth is all the rage, and actually a well-deserved one! Bone broth can boost your energy, diminish your cellulite, and shield you from colds and flu—even smooth out your wrinkles. Warm, rich bone broth has long been a go-to elixir for the ill. Humans have been sipping warm, rich bone broth since the beginnings of time, with early inns even offering a comforting cup to cold and weary travelers. Although bone broth's healing and nurturing properties have been recognized for millennia, its value in repairing the digestive tract, aiding detoxification, and reducing cellulite are more recent additions to its repertoire.

Bone broth might not be the first food that comes to mind when you think of beauty-enhancing foods, but perhaps it should be! As long as your broth is made from healthy animals (pasture-raised as opposed to factory-farmed), its powerful blend of minerals and other ultra-absorbable nutrients brings a flood of rejuvenation to your body. Broth contains radiance-boosting nutrients such as magnesium, potassium, amino acids, hyaluronic acid, and glycosaminoglycans, as well as gelatin, which is basically broken-down collagen. Collagen helps form elastin and other compounds responsible for your skin's youthful tone and texture. When your skin's collagen breaks down, cellulite and wrinkles become more noticeable. Bone broth not only helps reduce cellulite but can reverse the signs of aging, restoring skin's elasticity, hydration, and tone.

Cellulite also worsens when your body holds on to toxins, because toxins are stored in fat. Toxins in subcutaneous fat damage the skin's architecture, giving rise to those annoying lumps and bumps. Therefore, cellulite may be a sign that your detoxification mechanisms are underperforming. This is where bone broth's other magic comes in—it builds and strengthens the lining of your digestive tract to better absorb nutrients, remove toxins, and expel waste so that fewer toxins make it into your tissues.

Bone broth is rich in sulfur, potassium, and glycine, which support cellular and liver detoxification. Sulfur is the main ingredient in glutathione, your body's "master antioxidant" that plays a critical role in eliminating fat-soluble toxins. Some of the essential minerals in bone broth also act like chelators, preventing heavy metals from attaching to mineral receptor sites.

Bone broth's proteins and amino acids (collagen, gelatin, proline, glycine, glutamine, glucosamine, chondroitin, and others) help build strong muscles and connective tissue and reduce joint pain and inflammation, including pain related to arthritis. Penn State scientists found that athletes taking collagen supplements showed significant improvement in joint comfort and sports performance.

Due to its wealth of electrolytes, athletes have also used bone broth for electrolyte replacement after intense exertion, as well as accelerating healing after injuries. Electrolytes such as calcium, magnesium, potassium, phosphorous, and others support healthy circulation, proper nerve signaling, strong bones, and good digestive health.

The collagen and gelatin in bone broth can also tamp down inflammation in your gut, relieving gastrointestinal maladies such as irritable bowel syndrome, Crohn's disease, ulcerative colitis, and gastroesophageal reflux. Its glycine and glutamine are instrumental in reversing and preventing leaky gut. Bone broth helps resolve food allergies and fosters healthy gut flora, as well as showing great promise for combating autoimmune disorders. Whether you're superhealthy or challenged by ongoing health problems, bone broth is a fabulous addition to your overall nutrition program, and I've given it two thumbs up for all three phases of my New Fat Flush Plan.

Recommended Usage

- As a base for soups and stews, bone broth is beyond amazing. However, there are many other great uses such as to cook quinoa and other grains or to serve as a base for green drinks. With a little dash of salt, bone broth is a delicious beverage all by itself.
- Traditionally, people made bone broth from whatever was available at the time—beef, chicken, fish, lamb, or wild game. They used every part of the animal from the bones and marrow to the skin, feet, necks, tendons, and organs. Lengthy simmering over low heat causes the bones and connective tissues to break down and release their healing magic.
- Making your own bone broth is as easy as scoring some fresh, meaty bones—preferably including cartilaginous parts such as knuckles and chicken necks and feet—and then covering them with pure water.
- You can add whatever vegetables and herbs and spices you like—and then a healthy pinch of patience because you will then simmer and simmer and then simmer some more.

- Make sure your pot is full of bones with just enough water to cover—don't skimp on the bones. To fully extract their nutritional goodness, let your broth cook for 24 to 48 hours, depending on the size and type of bones. Adding a couple of tablespoons of vinegar to the water will help move the nutrients out of the bones and into your broth.
- You can source fresh bones from your local farmer or organic butcher, but carcasses from your roasted chickens and other meats will also work. A Thanksgiving turkey carcass makes a lovely turkey bone broth. Don't be afraid to mix and match your bones!
- If you're short on time, a number of companies are creating high-quality bone broths for delivery, typically in frozen form. Be very careful about your source! These broths should be made using only bones from 100 percent grass-fed (ideally pasture-raised) animals and organic vegetables and herbs, free of hormones, antibiotics, and artificial ingredients.
- A special Fat Flush bone broth is featured as part of my New Fat Flush Plan.

Just the Facts

- Bone broth is a prehistoric food dating back to the Stone Age. These broths have been used in Chinese medicine for 2,500 years for digestive health, building the blood, and strengthening the kidneys.
- In twelfth-century Egypt, a physician by the name of Moses Maimonides was said to prescribe chicken soup as a medicinal remedy for colds and asthma. This is likely the origin of what has come to be known as "Jewish penicillin."
- In the 1700s, enthusiasm over bone broth was reignited with "beef tea," a dilute, sepia-toned form of broth made by simmering rump meat and touted as a healthful beverage.
- Is chicken soup really an effective cold and flu remedy? Science says yes! Researchers found that people with respiratory infections who eat chicken soup experience a mild reduction in inflammation that actually does reduce their symptoms.

Boost the Benefits

- After your bone broth finishes cooking and cools, you may end up with a jiggly "meat Jell-O." Don't be alarmed—this is exactly what you want. The gelatin is a sign you did it right!
- Bone broth should keep in the refrigerator for three to four days or longer. In the freezer, it will last up to a year. If you freeze your broth in glass jars, make sure to leave plenty of air space to allow for the

expansion of the frozen liquid. This reduces the odds of the glass cracking. Make sure your broth is completely cool before freezing.
*   For added convenience, bone broth can be frozen in smaller quantities. Ice-cube trays and food-safe silicon trays specifically made for freezing baby food and other purees are handy for this purpose.

THINK TWICE!

*   *Making bone broth from the bones of conventionally farmed animals is at the very least counterproductive, but it may actually be harmful to your health. Animals exposed to contaminants in their food, water, and soil, such as heavy metals and pesticides, will concentrate these toxins in their bones. A small study looking at lead levels in chicken bone broth revealed that many contain several times the lead concentration of the water with which the broth was made. The cleaner your bones are, the better—whatever is in them (good and bad) will concentrate in your broth.*
*   *Do you know the difference between stock and bone broth? Once upon a time they were the same thing, but today stock can refer to anything in a cube, can, jar, or box—from bouillon powder to watered-down vegetable stock. Most of these commercial products are designed for flavor, not nutrition. Many include hydrolyzed protein, chemical additives, and emulsifiers that you're better off avoiding. One particularly bad additive is monosodium glutamate. MSG is a laboratory-concocted additive designed to "enhance" meat flavor, but it's a known neurotoxin.*

IT'S BEEN SAID . . .

Good broth will resurrect the dead.

SOUTH AMERICAN PROVERB

Nose-to-tail eating is the wisdom of our ancestors—we need to be eating all parts of the animal.

DR. KAAYLA DANIEL, THE NAUGHTY NUTRITIONIST

CHIA SEEDS

Fat Flush Factors

Blood Sugar Stabilizer
Cholesterol Zapper
Detoxifier
Energizer

Chia seeds are much more than the birth mother of chia pets! A concentrated source of protein, beneficial fats, fiber, vitamins, minerals, and antioxidants, chia can sustain your energy, sweep out your digestive tract, and keep you from moving down the path of type 2 diabetes. These tiny seeds pack twice the potassium of bananas and three times the antioxidant power of blueberries.

Chia are tiny seeds from the *Salvia hispanica* plant, which is a relative of mint. Native to South America, chia were an important food for the Aztecs and Mayans and prized for their energy-sustaining properties. In fact, the word *chia* is the ancient Mayan word for strength. Although they're grown mostly in Mexico and Bolivia, the United States began growing chia in 2014 due to their soaring popularity.

Chia are rich in both soluble and insoluble fiber and essential fats, offering a healthy omega-3 to omega-6 balance (30 percent omega-3, 40 percent omega-6). Chia's soluble fiber acts as a prebiotic, helping the good bacteria in your gut to fight off dangerous bacteria, viruses, yeasts, and other pathogens.

One of the things that make chia seeds so special is that they swell up like little balloons to 10 times their size, because their soluble fiber forms a gel when added to water. The benefit to you is that they slow down how quickly your body converts carbohydrates into sugar, keeping you feeling full longer, stabilizing your blood sugar, and keeping you hydrated as well as energized. This, along with their help for detox, aids in weight loss. Chia are also high in protein, and so they help build lean body mass.

Chia seeds nip cravings in the bud and may help trim off belly fat, which of course benefits your heart. Rat studies show chia seeds capable of lowering triglycerides, raising HDL, and reversing insulin resistance. A human study involving individuals with type 2 diabetes revealed that chia seeds can also lower blood pressure and tamp down inflammation.

When it comes to nutrient density, chia seeds are really remarkable! Just 1 ounce (about 2 tablespoons) packs 11 grams of fiber, 4 grams of protein, 9 grams of fat, and significant calcium, manganese, magnesium, and phosphorous—all for 137 calories. They also offer respectable amounts of zinc, niacin, potassium, thiamine, and vitamin B12. Because of their fat content, they help your body absorb the fat-soluble vitamins A, D, E, and K. Chia also contain a number of beneficial phytochemicals like caffeic acid and myricetin—as well as quercetin and kaempferol, known for their antioxidant, anti-inflammatory, and anticancer properties.

Along with flax and hemp seeds, chia seeds are an easy way to ramp up your nutritional intake. Just sprinkle a few tablespoons on your eggs, salads, and veggies or add to your smoothies, and watch your energy soar.

Recommended Usage

- Unlike flax, which should be ground for optimal nutrient absorption, chia are easily absorbable in their whole form, making them easy and convenient to use.
- Chia can be eaten raw, soaked in juice or tea, added to smoothies, or sprinkled on salads, vegetables, and casseroles. They can also be added to baked goods. Their taste is rather bland, and so you can pretty much add them to anything!
- If you soak chia, they "sprout" and release the "enzyme inhibitors" they used to protect the seed, making them easier to digest and freeing up more of the nutrients.
- Chia seed pudding makes a delicious, nutritious breakfast. Many recipes can be found online, but the recipes are typically a blend of chia seeds, coconut milk (or tigernut milk or any nut or soy milk), vanilla, sweetener, cinnamon, dried fruit, and nuts. If you make it the night before, it will be all thick and yummy by morning.
- Use chia seeds in place of pectin to make your homemade jellies gel.
- Chia seeds can be used in place of bread crumbs to thicken meatballs and meatloaf or can be used as a breading for fish and chicken.

Just the Facts

- Because of their ability to absorb both water and fat, chia can be used to thicken sauces and even can be used as an egg substitute. For the egg substitute, mix one tablespoon of chia seeds with three tablespoons of water. After the mixture sits for a few minutes, you'll have a gel that can be used in place of eggs in a recipe.
- You can now buy drinks with chia seeds already in them!

Boost the Benefits

- Chia come in black and white varieties. Is there any nutritional difference? As it turns out, yes! Although they are highly similar, one study discovered that darker chia have one additional antioxidant over the lighter: quercetin. The black also scored a tad bit higher on the ORAC test, which measures antioxidant power.
- Chia have another unexpected benefit—they are extraordinarily shelf stable and very resistant to rancidity without expensive packaging. Chia seeds will last up to two years without refrigeration due to the high levels of antioxidants they contain, which prevent their fats from rancidity.
- Are you an athlete? Aztec runners used chia for endurance. Chia seed gel helps athletes stay hydrated, as well as providing extra protein. One 2011 study found that chia seeds improve exercise performance as much as a sports drink.

Fat Flush in Action

- An ancient way of using chia for appetite control is soaking the seeds in water to create a bulky gel, then consuming the gel before and between meals. This is reported to reduce food consumption by up to 50 percent, as well as slowing down digestion. Simply soak one cup of chia seeds in two cups of water for 12 hours. You can eat one-quarter cup to one cup daily, especially when you are concerned about overeating.

THINK TWICE!

- *Because chia seeds are sticky and swell up, they should be used cautiously with children, elderly, and anyone with a history of dysphagia (trouble swallowing). If a bolus of seeds gets stuck in your throat, they can quickly form a sticky ball that can partially block your esophagus, which could require medical treatment. Make sure they are consumed with plenty of water.*

Fat Flush Fun

- Remember those chia pets? Now you can eat your chia pet! Chia microgreens are supernutrient-dense and easy to grow—all you need is a shallow glass or ceramic dish with a cover. Just add water!
- In Mexico, chia seeds were so highly revered that they were used as currency.

COCONUTS AND COCONUT OIL

Fat Flush Factors
Blood Sugar Stabilizer
Cholesterol Zapper
Energizer
Thermogenic

The health benefits of coconuts and coconut oil have really come to light over the past decade. From fueling your brain to boosting your metabolism to supporting your immune health, coconuts win the gold. About 80 percent of coconut meat is fat, and of that, 92 percent is saturated fat—and the kind you want.

Not all coconut oils are created equal. The natural, unrefined variety available today in nutrition stores is vastly different from the ultrarefined, deodorized, and bleached coconut oil poured into junk food in the 1980s, which was a cardiovascular nightmare. When we talk about the benefits of coconut oil, we are definitely not talking about that.

Populations for whom coconut is a dietary staple have far lower rates of cardiovascular disease and brain disease than Westerners. Vascular disease is a rarity among Polynesians; and the Kitevan people of New Guinea, who are also major coconut consumers, have extremely low to nonexistent coronary artery disease, sudden death, stroke, and brain disease. Coconuts and coconut oil may offer protection against brain disorders such as epilepsy and Alzheimer's disease. In a 2015 study, Alzheimer's patients given 40 milliliters of extra virgin coconut oil daily showed significantly improved cognition.

Coconut oil is about two-thirds medium-chain fatty acids, also known as medium-chain triglycerides, or MCTs. MCTs are metabolized by the body more like carbohydrates than long-chain triglycerides (LCTs), which are more common. Coconut and MCTs provide abundant energy without any of the insulin-related problems associated with high carbohydrate consumption.

LCTs (12 to 18 carbons long) are the predominant form of fat in the American diet, but MCTs (6 to 10 carbons long) have several unique nutritional advantages. MCTs go straight to your liver where they are used immediately for energy or turned into ketones. Ketogenic diets are beneficial for preventing and treating cancer. MCTs suppress appetite, stabilize blood sugar, raise HDL, and improve the overall lipid profile, while encouraging the shedding of excess body fat. MCTs have appetite-suppressing effects as well as help reduce visceral fat.

Coconuts and coconut oil contain an abundance of antioxidants and so can be regarded as antiaging foods. They also boost thyroid function, improve digestion and absorption of fat-soluble vitamins, and promote conversion of cholesterol into pregnenolone, which is a precursor to many important hormones. But the benefits don't stop there!

Fifty percent of the fat in coconuts is a type rarely found in nature called lauric acid. Your body converts lauric acid into the monoglyceride monolaurin, which is a boon to your immune system. Monolaurin has antiviral, antibacterial, antifungal, and antiprotozoal properties, effectively killing everything from *Candida albicans* to athlete's foot to head lice.

When it comes to coconuts, what's not to love?

Recommended Usage

- Not only is coconut oil a food, but it has numerous other applications. It makes an excellent moisturizer, deep hair conditioner, deodorant, and makeup remover.
- Try coconut oil for shaving your legs—use one teaspoon of oil per leg.
- Due to its antibacterial properties, coconut oil is excellent for oil pulling. For use as a toothpaste, add a little baking soda and peppermint oil.
- Coconut oil has some insect-repelling properties, which can be augmented by adding certain essential oils that bugs hate.
- Using a hand mixer, you can whip coconut oil into a luxurious body butter.
- Apply coconut oil to your scalp to control dandruff or itchiness.
- Coconut oil is excellent for chapped lips and for dry cuticles, heels, and elbows. It helps breastfeeding moms with cracked nipples and also works on puppy paws and baby bottoms.

Just the Facts

- Massaging babies with coconut oil has been shown to have health benefits, such as encouraging neonatal weight gain.
- Coconut oil can also be used as a diaper cream and as a treatment for cradle cap.

Boost the Benefits

+ When shopping for fresh coconut, coconut oil, or coconut milk, always select products that are as fresh and close to nature as possible. Certified organic, non-GMO is always preferable.

Fat Flush in Action

+ If you dislike the taste of coconut, use MCT oil, which is tasteless and has all the benefits of coconut oil.
+ Coconut oil's melting point is 78 degrees Fahrenheit. Below that it remains a solid.
+ For accuracy, measure solid or chilled coconut oil by spooning it into a measuring cup, packing it down, and then scraping over the top to level it, just as you would measure flour.
+ The smoke point for coconut oil is 350 degrees Fahrenheit, so it's not suitable for high-temperature cooking.

Be a Fat Flush Cook

+ Try drizzling coconut oil over the top of cooked veggies, meats, or fish.
+ Add coconut oil to oatmeal and soups for luscious nondairy creaminess.
+ Add coconut, coconut oil, or coconut milk (or MCT oil) to smoothies.
+ Add coconut oil (or MCT oil) to your morning coffee for a brain boost.
+ Add coconut flakes (unsweetened) to healthy nuts, seeds, and dried fruit for a delicious trail mix.
+ Coconut oil is an excellent fat for baked goods and for gentle stovetop cooking (not for high temperatures).
+ Try gently sautéing bananas in coconut oil with nutmeg, ginger, and cinnamon and serve over coconut milk "ice cream" for a luscious dessert.

THINK TWICE!

• *Keep your coconut oil out of direct sunlight.*

Fat Flush Fun

* Want to tackle a fresh coconut without losing a finger? Here is how, using nothing more than a chef's knife, butter knife, and vegetable peeler:
  - Working over a bowl and using a chef's knife (or a cleaver), carefully whack the coconut around its equator using the *blunt* side of the blade. Once the coconut breaks in half, continue hitting it to break it into smaller pieces. Now, using the butter knife, gently pry the flesh away from the shell—it usually comes off fairly easily. Then simply peel the brown skin off the flesh using your vegetable peeler. You now have the makings for homemade coconut milk or any other desired use. The taste of freshly harvested coconut is guaranteed to rock your world!

CRANBERRIES

Fat Flush Factors
Cholesterol Zapper
Detoxifier
Diuretic

Native to North America, the cranberry can still be found growing wild in the cool, sandy bogs of Massachusetts and New Jersey. It was Dutch and German settlers who named this bright-red berry, calling it "crane" berry after the bird-like shape of its blossoms.

Cranberries—and pure, unsweetened cranberry juice—enjoy superstar status as a prime component of the New Fat Flush Plan. Cranberries contain significant amounts of both flavonoids and polyphenolic compounds, shown to prevent the oxidation of LDL cholesterol. LDL cholesterol is the "bad" type of cholesterol, which becomes dangerous to the body only after it has been oxidized. Ongoing research continues to suggest that cranberries offer a natural defense against atherosclerosis and heart disease. At the Technical University of Denmark, researchers compared the health benefits of cranberry and blueberry juice. The results? Cranberries won, hands down. In fact, while cranberry juice proved to be a powerful antioxidant, blueberry juice served up no more nutritional benefit than sugar water.

Only a few years ago, some doctors discounted cranberry juice as a natural prevention for bladder infections. Now, thanks to research conducted by the Harvard Medical School and Rutgers University, physicians know that cranberries help prevent the bacteria *E. coli* from sticking to the lining of the bladder. The news gets even better. It turns out that cranberries have a similar effect in the mouth, preventing bacteria from gathering on the surface of your teeth where it can cause gingivitis and periodontal disease. The antibacterial power of cranberries also shows up in the stomach, providing much-needed protection against the ulcer-causing bacterium *H. pylori*.

All these health improvements make cranberries worth every penny. However, Fat Flushers know that cranberries offer another very important side effect. Pure cranberry juice is absorbed immediately into the system, where it helps keep your liver's detoxification pathways open; provides antioxidants called phenols, along with vitamin C–related bioflavonoids to strengthen your connective tissue; and based on my observations over the past 15 years, acts as a digestive aid for any stubborn fat deposits remaining in your lymphatic system. This could well be the reason why people on the Fat Flush Plan see their cellulite disappear.

So expand your consumption of cranberries *beyond* the Thanksgiving holiday, and you'll gain an abundance of health—and beauty—benefits all year long.

Recommended Usage

One cup of 100 percent pure, unsweetened cranberry juice per day.

Just the Facts

- In colonial times, cranberries did triple duty as a medicine, a colorful natural dye, and a symbol of peace.
- Cranberries are one of only three original American fruits still being produced today, with nearly 600 million pounds harvested every October. If you strung together all the cranberries produced in North America last year, they would stretch from Boston to Los Angeles more than 565 times!
- Cranberries are considered a "functional" food, meaning they provide natural health benefits far beyond basic nutrition.
- Based on serving size, pure, unsweetened cranberry juice has the highest antioxidant level of any cranberry product.
- Cranberry juice helps prevent a vitamin B12 deficiency by increasing the body's absorption of this important nutrient.

Boost the Benefits

- When shopping for cranberries, look for fruit that is shiny and plump and has a bright color. A good-quality, ripe cranberry will bounce.
- You may store cranberries in the refrigerator in their original, unopened plastic bags for one or two months. They may be kept frozen for eight to nine months. Once cooked, they will stay fresh for up to a month in a covered container in the refrigerator.
- Because overcooking gives them a bitter taste, cranberries should be cooked only until they "pop."

THINK TWICE!

- *When buying cranberry juice, remember to read labels carefully. The wording on the label provides strong clues to the content. For example, a cranberry "drink" or "cocktail" usually contains ample* amounts of sugar water or corn syrup, with a little real juice thrown in for good measure. Bottles marked "no sugar added" are often sweetened with apple or grape juice. For maximum fat-flushing benefit, look for 100 percent pure, unsweetened cranberry juice.

IT'S BEEN SAID . . .

For my entire life, my thighs bulged out at the sides. . . . I was the ultimate pear shape. Now my sides are straight and firm. I've been dieting off and on ever since I was in junior high, and this has never *happened before. I believe it's the daily cranberry juice mixed with water that helps the most. I could tell a real difference even in the first week or two of drinking it, and now if I get little or no cran-water when I travel, I really miss that cleaned-out leaner feeling I get while I'm drinking it.*

KATHY J., NEW YORK

FLAXSEED OIL

> ## Fat Flush Factors
>
> *Blood Sugar Stabilizer*
> *Cholesterol Zapper*
> *Detoxifier*
> *Energizer*

For Fat Flushers, flaxseed oil is a key element, capable of setting off a domino effect of weight loss and health benefits. It contains omega-3 (essential fatty acids), which, along with CLA (conjugated linoleic acid) and GLA (gamma-linolenic acid), are the missing links to health, beauty, and weight loss. As their name implies, essential fatty acids are vital for human health, but because they cannot be made by the body, they must be obtained from foods. If your waistline is expanding, it could be because of a deficiency in the right kind of fat!

An omega-3 deficiency promotes weight gain in several ways. First, the appetite center in your brain may not be getting the message that you are full, so you eat more than you need. Second, your metabolism slows down, causing you to take in more calories than you burn off. By consuming flaxseed oil, you'll feel full for up for three or four hours so you won't be tempted to overeat between meals. Also, the omega-3s in the flaxseed oil are known to boost serotonin levels in the brain. As a result, you won't feel depressed, and you won't feel the need to eat to release anxiety and stress. And flaxseed oil revs up your metabolism, stimulates bile production, and attracts oil-soluble toxins that have been lodged in fatty tissues in the body, eliminating them from your system.

Beyond being a dieter's dream, flaxseed oil plays a critical role in healthy brain function, proper thyroid and adrenal activity, and balanced hormones. It strengthens the immune system, helps maintain healthy blood and nerves, and breaks down cholesterol. The omega-3s in flaxseed oil are also needed to produce flexible cell membranes, which allow for efficient use of insulin and stabilization of blood sugar. In the colon, omega-3 fats help protect colon cells from cancer-causing toxins and free radicals, thus reducing the risk of colon cancer. And on the beauty front, flaxseed oil promotes glowing skin, shiny hair, and strong nails.

You can see why I consider flaxseed oil so vital to everyone's health and wellness. Is it any wonder that this precious oil has been nicknamed "liquid gold"? Do yourself a favor—get over your fear of fat and add flaxseed oil to your daily diet. You'll pare off the pounds and develop that Fat Flush "glow"!

Recommended Usage

Two tablespoons of flaxseed oil per day.

Just the Facts

- Flax plants grow well in most climates, except for areas with searing hot or bitterly cold weather.
- After settling in North America, most colonists made planting flax a top priority.
- For centuries, freshly pressed flaxseed oil was sold by street vendors in northern Europe.
- Dry skin is the first—and most common—sign that you are deficient in omega-3 fatty acids.

Boost the Benefits

- Flaxseed oil is highly perishable and should be purchased in opaque bottles that have been kept refrigerated.
- Because heat destroys the sensitive fatty acids in flaxseed oil, you cannot cook or bake with it. Avoid direct exposure to heat.
- Fresh flaxseed oil has a sweet, nutty flavor. It can vary from brand to brand, so be sure to try several to find the one that suits you best.
- By blending flaxseed oil with other foods, rather than taking it alone by the spoonful, you allow it to emulsify, which ensures better absorption of the essential fatty acids.

Be a Fat Flush Cook

- Add a tablespoon of flaxseed oil to your breakfast smoothie. Your appetite will be satisfied for hours!
- Mix yogurt and flaxseed oil for a healthy alternative to mayonnaise.
- For people on the New Fat Flush Plan, butter is a phase 3 treat. To give your phase 3 butter a bigger nutritional bite, try making a flavorful flax spread. Melt a stick of butter and remove it from the heat. Add four ounces of flaxseed oil and stir until blended. Pour the mixture into a container, cover it, and store in the refrigerator until it solidifies.
- For a great phase 3 snack, mix one tablespoon of flaxseed oil into a cup of yogurt and add your favorite fruit.

- Drizzle flaxseed oil over steamed veggies and then sprinkle with your favorite herbs. In fact, flaxseed oil may be added to any food after the food has been heated.

THINK TWICE!

- *If flaxseed oil tastes harsh, is intensely bitter, or feels scratchy to your throat, it is old and should be discarded.*

FLAX SEEDS

> ## Fat Flush Factors
>
> *Blood Sugar Stabilizer*
> *Cholesterol Zapper*
> *Detoxifier*

One of people's earliest food supplies, flax seeds definitely live up to their Latin name, *Linum usitatissium*, which means "most useful." These tiny brown seeds may not look like much, but they are held dear by Fat Flushers all over the globe for their omega-3 content and exceptional health benefits.

Slightly larger than sesame seeds, flax seeds taste sweet and somewhat nutty. They contain 40 percent oil and are the number one source of alpha-linolenic acid, an essential fatty acid required for efficient metabolism. Flax seeds are also a superior source of lignans, plant estrogens known for their ability to fight cancer, keep viruses at bay, and balance hormone levels. Ounce for ounce, flax seeds contain 800 times as many lignans as any other plant.

Lignan-rich flax seeds have also been shown to reduce insulin resistance, which, in turn, has a positive impact on estrogen levels and breast cancer risk. And since insulin resistance is an early warning sign for type 2 diabetes, flax seeds may also provide protection against this disease, which is currently a U.S. epidemic.

When flax seeds come in contact with a liquid, they become soft and jelly-like, making them highly useful as an intestinal cleanser and bowel regulator. The *soluble* fiber in flax seeds helps reduce the amount of carbohydrates absorbed by our bodies. In addition, the fiber stabilizes blood sugar levels, minimizes cholesterol absorption, and lowers cholesterol levels. And the five grams of *insoluble* fiber per tablespoon helps ease elimination by absorbing water in the intestinal tract. In addition, flax seeds contain prussic acid, which improves digestion. Be sure to take advantage of the healthy "scrubbing action" this Fat Flush superfood has to offer!

Recommended Usage

Two tablespoons of ground flax seeds per day.

Just the Facts

- Currently, Canada is the major producer of flax seeds.
- The only difference between brown and golden flax seeds is their color.
- As a source of plant sterols, flax seeds boost the immune function.

Boost the Benefits

- You may purchase flax seeds either whole or already ground. While ground flax seeds may be more convenient, whole flax seeds have a longer shelf life.
- Whole flax seeds can be found in prepackaged containers as well as in bulk bins. If you purchase them from a bulk bin, make sure the bin is covered and has no signs of moisture.
- Don't consume whole flax seeds, or you'll miss out on important nutrients. The lignans are found in the fibrous shell hull of the flax seeds and are only released when the seeds are ground.
- If you purchase whole flax seeds, store them in an airtight container in a dark, dry, cool place, where they should maintain their freshness for several months.
- Packages of preground flax seeds should be vacuum-packed and/or refrigerated, because at room temperature, ground flax seeds spoil within just a few days.
- If you grind flax seeds at home, keep them in a tightly sealed container in the refrigerator or freezer to prevent them from becoming rancid.
- To extend the freshness, you may freeze both whole and ground flax seeds for up to 1 year.
- To grind whole flax seeds, try a coffee or seed grinder. You'll have beautifully ground flax seeds at the push of a button!

Be a Fat Flush Cook

- Sprinkle ground flax seeds onto a variety of foods, from yogurt to salads to steamed veggies to a bowl of soup.
- Add flax seeds to your homemade muffin, cookie, or bread recipes. But remember not to set your oven temperature higher than 350 degrees.
- To pump up the nutritional volume of your breakfast shake, add ground flax seeds.
- To give sliced fruit a nuttier flavor, sprinkle some ground flax seeds on top of it.

THINK TWICE!

- *Flax seeds contain cyanogenic glycosides, naturally occurring plant compounds, which, in large amounts, can suppress the thyroid's ability to take up sufficient iodine. To deactivate the glycosides, toast your whole flax seeds for 15 minutes in a 250 degree oven prior to grinding them.*

IT'S BEEN SAID . . .

Every morning and every evening, I mix ground flax seeds, unsweetened cranberry juice, and water to make a Fat Flush Long Life Cocktail. I love the nutty flavor of the flax seeds, and it's great knowing that something so simple is working to improve my health!

DEBBIE R., IDAHO

HEMP SEEDS

Fat Flush Factors
Blood Sugar Stabilizer
Cholesterol Zapper
Detoxifier
Energizer

Hemp seeds are one of nature's greatest gifts, perfect little bundles of benefits for your entire body. They're about one-third healthful fats and one-quarter protein, as well as a magnificent source of natural gamma-linolenic acid. You also can't get much better than hemp seeds for their 3 to 1 omega-3 to omega-6 ratio. Overall, these little dynamos can sustain energy, encourage weight loss, reduce food cravings, lower blood pressure, improve blood sugar and lipid profiles, and tamp down inflammation.

GLA—also found in borage, evening primrose, and black currant seed oils—supports the normal growth and function of your cells, nerves, muscles, and organs. GLA also happens to be the "good omega-6" known for flushing away body fat, a blessing for those wishing to shed a little excess padding. GLA is an essential fatty acid that triggers fat burning instead of fat storage by boosting your metabolism in a couple of ways, including actually "using up" a lot of calories. GLA is also a natural hormone-balancing fat that can reduce PMS and menopausal symptoms.

If you have an optimally healthy body, you can synthesize GLA from linoleic acid, found in certain oils, grains, and seeds. But due to a number of common dietary and lifestyle factors in today's society, most of our bodies don't make that conversion.

Hemp belongs to the genus *Cannibis sativa*, cultivated for thousands of years for everything from nutrient-rich seeds and oils to industrial fiber, paper, textiles, building materials, and even fuel. In the United States, the nutritional benefits of hemp seeds have been all but ignored due to their botanical relationship with the drug and medicinal varieties of *Cannabis*. Although hemp and marijuana come from the same plant species, there are notable differences. Please don't be confused—hemp seeds are simply incapable of producing a psychotropic reaction because their THC (tetrahydrocannabinoid) content is so low.

THC is the compound in marijuana responsible for inducing the "high." Hemp contains only a trace of THC (0.3 to 1.5 percent), and most of it is in the hull of the seed. The majority of hemp seeds produced for consumption are actually "hemp hearts," which have had their hulls removed, reducing their THC even further.

Getting back to hemp seeds' nutritional properties, their protein is substantial—equal to that of beef or lamb but in a more digestible, bioavailable form. It's also a complete protein, providing all the essential amino acids. Just 30 grams of hemp seeds (2 to 3 tablespoons) contains 11 grams of protein. Hemp seeds offer significant amounts of the amino acids methionine and cysteine, as well as very high levels of arginine and glutamic acid. Arginine lowers blood pressure by relaxing your blood vessels. There is also evidence that hemp seeds may decrease clot formation and speed up recovery after a heart attack.

The fiber in hemp seeds is contained mostly in the hull, so hemp hearts contain relatively little fiber. However, what they lack in fiber they make up for in calcium, magnesium, iron, manganese, phosphorous, potassium, zinc, and vitamins A, B1, B2, B3, B6, D, and E.

Hemp seeds also appear to have strong anti-inflammatory benefits, most likely related to their generous GLA. One study found that hemp seed GLA reduces symptoms by 25 percent for arthritis sufferers. Hemp seed contains plant sterols that may reduce your risk of colon and prostate cancer. New studies are emerging all the time, such as one that identified four compounds in hemp seed (lignanamides) that show promise in protection from Alzheimer's disease. Finally, hemp seed has benefits for your skin, hair, and nails.

Hemp seeds are not a replacement for flax and chia seeds, but they're a great addition to them, bringing along their own unique nutritional properties. When it comes to hemp's health benefits, science has barely scratched the surface—I suspect many secrets await our discovery with this amazing superfood.

Recommended Usage

- Do not cook hemp seeds; eat them raw, because high temperatures will denature their delicate fats.
- Hemp seeds have a pleasantly nutty flavor, somewhat akin to walnut.
- You can sprinkle hemp seeds on just about anything—salads, veggies, quinoa, oatmeal, or even yogurt.
- Blend hemp hearts into your smoothie to bump up your protein and healthful fats.
- Hemp hearts can be blended with water to make hemp milk, which can be used as a dairy substitute like nut milks.

Just the Facts

• The United States is the world's largest consumer of hemp products; yet it is the only industrialized country that also outlaws their production. The cultivation of hemp was banned in 1970 when the federal Controlled Substances Act took effect. The law doesn't distinguish between marijuana the drug, marijuana the medicine, and hemp the food—despite major differences among them.

• Some hemp is being bred for high CBD content. CBD is cannabidiol, which has a multitude of health benefits. Since hemp is naturally low in THC, these medicinal hemp varieties are packed with powerful healing potential.

Boost the Benefits

• Due to the delicate fats in hemp seeds, they are prone to rancidity. If your hemp seeds have a funky taste or smell, discard them. The less heat and light they are exposed to, the better, so packages without a see-through window are preferable. They are often stored in the refrigerated section of food markets. Pay attention to "packaged on" or "best before" dates.

• Store hemp seeds in an airtight container in your refrigerator or freezer to extend their freshness. Once opened, a bag of hemp seeds will last about a year in the fridge or freezer or three to four months in your pantry.

• Hemp seed oil is also available, which can be helpful for skin disorders such as psoriasis, eczema, and dermatitis.

THINK TWICE!

• *Rancid GLA products are more likely to cause digestive upset, so again, if your hemp seeds smell "off," toss them and start anew.*

Fat Flush Fun

• The oldest known records of hemp farming date back 5,000 years in China, although hemp industrialization may date back to ancient Egypt.

• Hemp plants absorb four times more carbon dioxide than trees. Hemp has a very short growing cycle (12 to 14 weeks), which makes it a highly sustainable crop that can combat global warming.

• For thousands of years, 90 percent of all ships' ropes and sails were constructed from hemp—as were the first Bibles, maps, and flags as well as the first drafts of the Constitution and Declaration of Independence. Even the word *canvas* derives from hemp: the Middle English word *canevas* comes from the Latin word *cannabis.*

• In seventeenth- and eighteenth-century America, refusing to grow hemp was against the law. In Virginia between 1763 and 1769, you could be thrown in jail for refusing to grow hemp. Americans were allowed to pay taxes with hemp from 1631 until the early nineteenth century.

• Henry Ford's first Model T was constructed from hemp, as well as being fueled by hemp gasoline!

LEMONS

Fat Flush Factors
Cholesterol Zapper
Detoxifier
Diuretic
Thermogenic

Originally developed as a cross between a lime and a citron, lemons first appeared in China over 2,000 years ago. Christopher Columbus brought lemons to the Americas, and they have been grown in Florida ever since! Many people think of lemons only in terms of lemonade, but nutritionally this little yellow fruit can do much more than quench your thirst on a hot summer day.

Lemons are high in vitamin C, supplying four times more than oranges. As the primary water-soluble antioxidant in the body, vitamin C travels through your system, preventing cellular damage and cholesterol buildup by zapping any free radicals it meets. Recently, researchers discovered a substance in lemons called limonene. This essential oil has been shown to shrink cancerous tumors, detoxify carcinogens in the body, and stimulate the healthy flow of lymph fluids.

Lemons assist in the digestive process by producing necessary enzymes, invigorating the gallbladder and liver, and promoting the absorption of protein and minerals from foods. Lemon juice also helps liquefy fat so that it can be flushed out of your system faster. And as if that weren't enough, drinking lemon juice in hot water acts as a mild diuretic, ridding the body of retained water and toxins. It may also help to reduce cellulite by cleansing the lymphatic system and stimulating blood flow to the skin.

To top it off, lemons also provide small amounts of vitamin B6, potassium, calcium, magnesium, and folate. So run, don't walk, to pick up this Fat Flush superfood today!

Recommended Usage
The juice of at least one lemon every day.

Just the Facts

- Unlike oranges, lemons continue to ripen even after they are picked.
- Consuming lemons with sugar negates many of the health benefits of the fruit. The sugar lowers immunity, interferes with digestion, and leeches vitamins and minerals from the body.
- Aromatherapists believe that the smell of a lemon is beneficial because it helps reduce feelings of stress and boosts the immune system.
- Much of the taste and aroma of a lemon comes from the "zest"—oils that are abundant in the fruit's peel.

Boost the Benefits

- To find a good-quality lemon, remember that the thinner the skin, the more flesh the lemon will have—and the juicier it will be. Look for firm, fine-textured lemons that are heavy for their size.
- Pick lemons with a bright-yellow color, because the ones with a green tinge are not fully ripe and will be more acidic.
- Lemons are *overripe* if they are wrinkled, are reddish in color, or have soft or hard patches.
- If you plan to use the skin or zest of the lemon, choose fruit that is certified organic to avoid exposure to pesticides and wax.
- As long as they are protected from sunlight, lemons will stay fresh at room temperature for about one week.
- To keep lemons longer, store them in the refrigerator crisper where they will keep for about four weeks.
- Use a lemon as quickly as possible after cutting it.
- Since lemons produce more juice when they are warm, bring them to room temperature before juicing them by placing them in a bowl of warm water for several minutes. Rolling a lemon under the palm of your hand on a hard surface also produces more juice.
- Lemon juice can be frozen. Place freshly squeezed lemon juice in ice-cube trays until frozen. Then store the lemon cubes in plastic bags in the freezer until they are needed.

Be a Fat Flush Cook

- Combine lemon juice with olive oil or flaxseed oil, freshly crushed garlic, and cayenne to make a zesty salad dressing.
- Because acids help proteins coagulate, your poached eggs will keep their shape if you add a few drops of lemon juice to the cooking water.
- Squirt lemon juice on cut fruits or white vegetables to help them keep their color.

- When preparing fish, place thin lemon slices underneath and around the fish. As the fish bakes or broils, the lemon slices will soften and may be eaten along with the fish.
- That glass of water will have more zip and look prettier if you add a slice of lemon to it.

THINK TWICE!

- When preparing recipes that include lemons or lemon juice, use nonreactive cookware, such as stainless steel, enamel, or plastic. Exposing lemon to uncoated iron, copper, or aluminum cookware can discolor the food and leave a metallic taste.

IT'S BEEN SAID . . .

First, I learned to "lemonize" my foods. Now, I serve lemon wedges with all my meals. Squeezing lemon juice on my foods serves as a great salt substitute and really helps to cut the fat. Give it a try!

ELLEN H., NORTH CAROLINA

I come from a long line of cellulite-prone women, so you can imagine how happy I was to find a way to eliminate it! I figured that if the cellulite went away, any additional weight loss would be a bonus. The majority of my cellulite disappeared in the first two weeks of following the Fat Flush Plan, including the hot lemon water every morning. Even though I didn't get on a scale, I could see my thighs shrinking. I'm one happy woman!

CHARLI S., WASHINGTON

WATER

Fat Flush Factors
Detoxifier
Diuretic
Thermogenic

Did you know that the average person loses 10 cups of water each day just by breathing, perspiring, and using the bathroom? Yet a recent survey conducted by the International Bottled Water Association found that most Americans drink no more than five cups of water a day. While additional water is absorbed from the foods we eat, the math still doesn't add up, especially when many people counteract their intake of water by consuming caffeine-filled teas, coffees, or sodas, which inhibit the reabsorption of water. It's no wonder that a Cornell University survey showed that 75 percent of Americans are chronically dehydrated!

Even mild dehydration, such as a 2 percent drop in body water, can produce problems, including memory deficits, an inability to focus, and daytime fatigue. Some subtle signs of dehydration include dry lips, dark-colored urine, muscle or joint soreness, headaches, crankiness, fatigue, and constipation. Ironically, if you don't drink enough water, your body senses trouble and begins to hang on to every bit of water it can. If you fail to hydrate your body, it stores water between cells and you end up carrying excess water weight.

To make matters worse, if you are dehydrated, your body stores more fat. Why? Without water, your kidneys are forced to call on the liver to help perform their functions. This keeps the liver from being able to burn as much fat as it normally would, so the fat gets deposited—often around the belly. In addition to reducing fat deposits and ridding the body of toxins, consuming generous amounts of water is an effective way to reduce cravings. Because water is a natural appetite suppressant and helps you feel full, you may not feel hungry if you drink it regularly throughout the day.

Still not convinced? Keep in mind that water is a powerful tool for a clear, beautiful complexion. Your body prioritizes where the water goes, and since vital organs take precedence, your skin is last on the list. If you fail to drink enough water, your skin will suffer more than any other part of your body. Being well hydrated also helps reduce constipation and, because water allows for efficient elimination, has even been shown to decrease the risk of colon cancer by 45 percent. Furthermore, a 2002 study concluded that a daily intake of at least five glasses of water cut the risk of heart disease in half! So "Bottoms up" to all my Fat Flush friends.

Recommended Usage

Eight 8-ounce glasses of water per day (which can be enjoyed in your cran-water or tea or coffee) plus one 8-ounce glass for each hour of light activity and even more if you speak a great deal, which surprisingly creates dehydration.

Just the Facts

- The human body is nearly 70 percent water. This amount can be seriously affected by stress, alcohol, and caffeine.
- While people can live without food for about a month, they can't last a week without water.
- If you wait until you are thirsty to drink some water, you will already be dehydrated! By the time you feel thirsty, you have already lost over 1 percent of your total body water.

Boost the Benefits

- Keep a bottle of water with you in the car so that you can grab a few sips while you're on the run.
- Don't drink ice water with meals, as it dilutes digestive enzymes. To enhance digestion, enjoy a cup of hot water with lemon immediately after your meal.
- Caffeinated coffees, teas, and sodas are no substitute for water, since caffeine functions as a diuretic, causing you to lose water through frequent urination.
- Because your body loses water while you sleep, it's a great idea to start and end your day with a glass of water.
- Keep drinking while you exercise! By replacing the fluid you lose as sweat, water keeps your energy level stable during exercise. Since water plays an important role in the transport of nutrients and chemical reactions in the body, staying hydrated boosts your metabolism, increasing the number of calories burned during daily activities. So have a bottle of water handy and take frequent water breaks.

Be a Fat Flush Cook

- Adding ice cubes to your morning smoothie creates a thick drink with the power to hydrate.

- Make water-filled foods a regular part of your diet. These include broth-based soups, lettuce, broccoli, and citrus fruits.
- Wean yourself off regular juice by diluting it with water, adding less and less juice as time goes on.
- To entice yourself (and your family members) to drink more water, try some of the following tips:
    - Add a splash of lemon juice to your water for a tangy flavor.
    - Make juice cubes by filling an ice-cube tray with lemon or cranberry juice. Pop a cube or two into a tall glass of water for a refreshing, festive drink.
    - Drop a couple of frozen strawberries into your water.

2 Fat Flush Proteins

The human organism needs an ample supply of good building material to repair the effects of daily wear and tear.

—INDRA DEVI, YOGA TEACHER AND WRITER

"Vegetarian/vegan sources are the best source of protein; no, animal foods are." "We all need more protein; no, we really need less." Sound familiar? There is probably no food group more controversial than protein these days. The truth is that there is no source of protein that works for everybody, but the good news is that Fat Flush contains them all—whey, pea and rice, beans, beef, poultry, fish, lamb, and eggs.

Composed of amino acids, protein is vital as a "building block" for every human cell. It also maintains proper fluid balance, supports hormone and enzyme development, enhances the immune system, and, of course, provides energy to every part of the body. Since our bodies can't store protein, it must be supplied on a daily basis from the foods we eat—whether that be vegan or derived from animals.

Unfortunately, many people have a media-driven fear of fat, which extends to a fear of eating certain proteins. You needn't worry that any of my Fat Flush protein selections presented in this chapter will hinder your health or weight loss. For example, beef is included as a Fat Flush superfood because it is the highest dietary source of L-carnitine, an incredibly effective fat-burning nutrient. And eggs have been found innocent of raising cholesterol levels. In fact, the *Journal of the American Medical Association* published results of an eight-year study that tracked nearly 40,000 men and 80,000 women and showed there was no link between egg consumption and the risk of coronary heart disease.

The protein-rich Fat Flush superfoods found in this chapter are important weight loss tools. Adding more—not less—protein to your diet makes great dietary sense, especially if you are extremely active, to help rebuild muscle tissues (I'm talking about at least 45 minutes of moderate exercise four to five times weekly). Consuming adequate protein is also crucial to warding off osteoporosis as we get older—at least 20 to 30 grams per meal, which is exactly the Fat Flush Rx.

Protein helps you feel full faster and requires more energy to digest than other foods, thereby using up more calories and contributing to weight loss. In fact, by building muscle mass, protein has been shown to raise your metabolism by nearly 30 percent, which gears up your calorie-burning thyroid gland. By slowing down the absorption of glucose into the bloodstream, protein stabilizes your blood sugar level. And as you flush more and more fat, protein-rich foods will help preserve your all-important lean muscle tissue. Think of protein as your supersculptor hunger buster.

BEANS

Fat Flush Factors
Blood Sugar Stabilizer
Cholesterol Zapper
Detoxifier
Energizer

Beans are a Fat Flush food because they have a unique combination of fiber and protein that fills you up, decreases your appetite, and helps you eat less overall. A 2014 meta-analysis found that people who consumed a cup of beans felt 31 percent fuller than those who didn't.

There are literally thousands of varieties of beans! For this discussion, however, we're talking about common beans—the edible dried seeds in the legume family (black, pinto, kidney, navy, garbanzo, and the like). These are beans whose seeds are eaten, but not the pods, and not those classified as peas or lentils (which are also legumes). Common beans come from the *Phaseolus vulgaris* species.

The primary health benefits of beans come from their powerful blend of protein and fiber. A typical 1-cup serving of cooked beans provides a whopping 15 grams of fiber and 15 grams of protein—a dose of protein equal to 2 ounces of meat, fish, or poultry. It's very rare, if not unheard of, to find this combination of fiber and protein in any other food, which is why they're included in my New Fat Flush Plan.

Beans have been shown to provide benefits for your heart and digestive systems, and they're dynamite for blood sugar regulation, which reduces your risk for type 2 diabetes. In terms of preventing diabetes, research is focusing in on the alpha-amylase inhibitory effects of beans whose naturally occurring compounds slow down the activity of alpha-amylase enzymes. These enzymes are key in breaking down starch into sugar, which is why, in addition to their fiber, beans are so helpful with blood sugar regulation.

Any vegetarian knows that the amino acid profiles of beans and grains combine to form a complete protein. However, beans on their own supply several important vitamins and minerals such as molybdenum, folate, copper, manganese, vitamin B1, phosphorous, iron, magnesium, calcium, and zinc. Calcium and phosphorus are important for your bone structure, while iron and zinc help maintain the strength and elasticity of your bones and joints.

Black beans have an added nutritional kick because their dark outer seed coat is rich in three anthocyanin flavonoids: delphinidin, petunidin, and malvidin. They also contain two other flavonoids, kaempferol and quercetin, as well as saponins, hydroxycinnamic acids (ferulic, sinapic, and chlorogenic acid), and many triterpenoids—all fancy names for botanical compounds that do a number of good things in your body!

Quercetin is an anti-inflammatory antioxidant that protects your heart by reducing atherosclerosis and shielding you from damage by LDLs. Saponins optimize your lipids and protect your cardiovascular system, in addition to preventing cancer cells from multiplying and spreading. In addition to beans' fiber content, their saponin may help explain why those who eat beans several times per week are less likely to develop colorectal polyps and colon cancer.

Indigestible fiber is particularly high in black beans, which provides the perfect substrate for good bacteria to thrive in your colon—particularly the ones that produce butyric acid, which your intestinal lining requires for proper function. The fiber and protein in beans make them hearty, keeping you feeling fuller longer, helping you consume less, and promoting regular bowel movements. Beans are just a great all-around food, and you can add them in phase 3 of my New Fat Flush Plan.

Recommended Usage

- Unlike most canned vegetables that have lost much of their nutritional value, canned beans retain most of their nutrients and are nutritionally comparable to those you cook yourself. However, you still need to be careful about beans from cans lined with resin-based can liners that use bisphenol A (BPA). There is some evidence that other plastics—even those listed as BPA-free—may leach into the food. The safest way is to cook your beans from scratch in order to avoid all the plastics.
- If you do used canned beans, select varieties with no added sodium, and make sure to drain and rinse them thoroughly.
- When using dried beans, it's important to sort through them for any small rocks or other debris that may have made their way into the package. Rinse and soak dried beans in water for at least 8 to 10 hours before cooking for the best flavor and texture.
- Whether we should use or discard the soaking water has been a matter of much debate over the years, but I think the discarders have won. Getting rid of the soaking water means flushing out some of the phytates and tannins that may compromise nutrient bioavailability, as well as reducing flatulence-inducing compounds. You can tell beans are adequately soaked when they split easily between your fingers. Soaking dried beans also reduces their cooking time.

• Try adding beans to soups, grain dishes, or salads, or grind the beans into hummus. Hummus can be made from many different beans—not just garbanzos!

Just the Facts

• Legumes were among our first cultivated crops. Archaeologists have carbon-dated peas back to 9750 BC. Other evidence suggests that native peoples of Mexico and Peru were cultivating bean crops in 7000 BC. Chickpeas, lentils, and fava beans have been found in Egyptian tombs dating back more than 4,000 years.
• Today's "common beans" originated in Central and South America. In the fifteenth century, Spanish explorers returning from the New World introduced beans to Europe, which were then spread to Africa and Asia by Spanish and Portuguese traders.
• Today, beans are grown on every continent except Antarctica. Brazil and India are the largest commercial producers, turning out almost 18 million metric tons of dried beans annually. Brazil grows more black beans than any other country.
• Adzuki beans have the highest level of protein of just about any bean variety. And one cup of cooked chickpeas gives you as much potassium as a small banana.
• Beans are a rich source of the trace mineral molybdenum, an integral component of the enzyme sulfite oxidase, which is responsible for detoxifying sulfites.

Boost the Benefits

• Dried beans stored in an airtight container in a cool, dry, and dark place will keep up to 12 months.
• "Beans, beans, the musical fruit—the more you eat, the more you toot!" There's so much truth in that little jingle! The consumption of beans and other legumes is known to cause many people to have gas. Legumes contain oligosaccharides known as galactans, complex sugars that the body can't digest, as it lacks the enzyme alpha-galactosidase. If you experience bean-induced flatulence, there are some things you can do.
• Try introducing beans into your diet in smaller quantities. Gradually increase your consumption of them—meaning eat smaller quantities more often. As previously discussed, try soaking your dried beans before cooking them. You may wish to soak them for longer, which makes for sprouted beans—just make sure you drain and discard that soaking water. Some people report that adding coriander or cumin during cooking also helps reduce gassiness.

Fat Flush in Action

- Adding salt, sugar, or acidic foods (like tomatoes) to your dried beans may harden them and result in longer cooking times.
- Canned beans are fully cooked and need only be heated briefly (after thorough rinsing and draining) for hot recipes.

THINK TWICE!

- *A lectin called phytohaemagglutinin is present in many common bean varieties and is especially concentrated in red kidney beans. Lectins have some toxic effects in the body, as the plant produces them to protect itself and keep predators away. Evidence exists that lectins may promote leptin resistance.*
- *Many beans and other legumes have substantial amounts of naturally occurring compounds called oxalates. In certain medical conditions (kidney stones being one), oxalates and therefore beans must be restricted to prevent an overaccumulation inside the body.*

Fat Flush Fun

- Beans are a heliotropic plant, meaning the leaves tilt throughout the day to face the sun. At night, they go into a folded "sleep" position.

BEEF

Fat Flush Factors

Energizer
Thermogenic

For years, the media gave beef a bad rap, causing many people to shy away from buying even the leanest cuts of beef. Much to my delight, the current popularity of high-protein diets has boosted sales of beef across America; yet we still consume 25 percent less beef than we did in the mid-1970s. When was the last time you enjoyed some beef? I'm not talking about a fast-food hamburger, but rather a lean, tasty piece of steak, fillet, or roast. This nutrient-rich food promotes a strong immune system, provides energy to every cell, and helps build those all-important fat-burning muscles.

Beef is hearty and deeply flavored and ranks high as a source of protein, vitamin B12, zinc, and the potent fat-flushing fat-burner L-carnitine. A 3-ounce serving of beef supplies as much iron as 3 cups of raw spinach and as much zinc as 30 ounces of tuna. Beef also ranks high in iron, phosphorus, selenium, and the B-complex vitamins. In addition, about half the fat in beef is healthy monounsaturated fat, which does not raise cholesterol levels.

Beef's vitamin B12 content helps the body convert the potentially dangerous chemical homocysteine into harmless molecules, decreasing the risk of heart attack, stroke, and even osteoporosis. Organic beef is also a very good source of the trace mineral selenium, which helps reduce the risk of colon cancer and supports antioxidant activity in the liver and throughout the body. In addition, the zinc in lean beef helps prevent blood vessel damage that can lead to atherosclerosis and is also needed for proper functioning of the immune system.

Most of the beef available today is raised on grass and fattened on feedlots, with feed consisting of corn and molasses plus a hefty dose of antibiotics and other additives. For meat that is free of antibiotics, added hormones, and pesticides, consider buying organically certified beef. Another option is to look for grass-fed beef, which is rich in essential fatty acids, vitamin E, and beta-carotene. (You'll find an extensive list of grass-fed beef providers in my book *The New Fat Flush Plan*.) Grass-fed beef contains significant amounts of two "good" fats, monounsaturated oils and stearic acid, but no artificial trans fatty acids. Grass-fed beef is also the richest known natural source of CLA and is lower in total fat and calories than conventional beef.

Recommended Usage

Up to four 4-ounce servings per week.

Just the Facts

- At least a dozen cuts of beef are leaner than a skinless chicken thigh, including a sirloin steak, round steak, flank steak, tenderloin, tri-tip roast, and rump roast.
- Meat labeled "prime" is tender and juicy, but it is generally higher in fat than other grades of meat.
- A four-ounce serving of lean beef provides over 60 percent of the daily requirement for protein.
- A recent study published in the *Journal of Animal Science* concluded that a serving of grass-fed beef has less cholesterol than the same amount of chicken breast.

Boost the Benefits

- At the grocery store, make raw beef the last item added to your grocery cart. Put the meat packages in plastic bags to keep juices from dripping onto other foods.
- Always check the sell-by date on the label and choose the beef with the latest date.
- Look for beef with a bright-red color. Steaks and roasts should feel firm, not mushy.
- Go for the beef with the least amount of fat. Any fat on the meat should be white in color, not yellow, since meat with yellow fat is usually less tender.
- For the freshest and leanest ground beef, select a round or sirloin steak and ask the butcher to grind it for you.
- Refrigerate or freeze fresh beef immediately. Never leave beef sitting out at room temperature. Whole cuts of beef may be refrigerated in the coldest part of the refrigerator for three to five days, while refrigerated ground beef should be used within one or two days.
- To freeze beef, wrap it tightly in freezer paper. Ground beef should keep for about three months, and whole cuts are good for six months.
- Thaw frozen beef in the refrigerator or in cold water—never at room temperature. Likewise, you should marinate beef in the refrigerator, not on the counter.
- Food safety experts recommend using a thermometer to check for the "doneness" of cooked beef. The internal temperature of the meat should be at least 160 degrees.

THINK TWICE!

- *Always wash your hands thoroughly with hot soapy water after you handle raw beef.*
- *After handling raw beef, sanitize counters, cutting boards, and other surfaces with a solution of one teaspoon of chlorine bleach per quart of water.*
- *Discard beef that is beginning to smell or that you feel may be getting too old. Freezing it will not kill harmful bacteria.*

Be a Fat Flush Cook

- If you use grass-fed beef with its extremely low fat content, brush it with a bit of virgin olive oil to prevent drying and sticking. And keep in mind that it requires about 30 percent less cooking time than conventional beef.
- Sauté thin slices of steak or some lean ground beef in a bit of broth with onions and garlic. Add some no-salt tomato sauce or fresh tomatoes and serve over spaghetti squash.
- Skewer cubes of beef with your favorite Fat Flush vegetables. Brush with a little olive oil and grill.
- Thinly sliced cooked tenderloin makes for a wonderful sandwich. Top it with onion slices and a crisp leaf of romaine lettuce.
- Try a spice rub made up of your favorite Fat Flush herbs and spices. Just rub the mixture on the meat prior to cooking.
- After removing the cooked beef from the heat, let the cooked beef sit, covered and in a warm place, for about 10 minutes to allow the juices to redistribute.
- To preserve juiciness, avoid piercing the meat with a fork. Instead, always use tongs to turn your beef.

EGGS

Fat Flush Factors
Blood Sugar Stabilizer
Energizer

An egg is one of nature's most nutritious creations. Except for vitamin C, eggs provide a perfect balance of every important vitamin and mineral. In addition, eggs are protein-rich, inexpensive, and delicious. For many years, eggs got a bad rap because of their cholesterol content. Yet people who eat only egg whites and skip the yolks are really missing out. While it's true that the egg yolk contains all the fat, it also provides nearly half the protein and most of the vitamins. And while eggs are high in cholesterol, researchers have determined—in over 200 studies spanning the past 25 years—that it is not cholesterol but rather the amount of *saturated fat* in foods that affects cholesterol levels.

Recently, the "classic" egg has been improved upon, and we can now purchase eggs that have a higher content of omega-3, a polyunsaturated fatty acid known to reduce blood triglyceride levels and the risk of heart disease. Omega-3–enriched eggs come from hens that are fed a special diet of ground flax seeds, which are higher in omega-3 fatty acids and lower in saturated fatty acids than other grains.

In addition, eggs are a great source of choline, a key nutrient required for brain function and nervous system health. Choline also affects cardiovascular health since it helps convert harmful homocysteine molecules into a benign substance. Eggs also contain a hefty supply of biotin, a B vitamin involved in producing energy by metabolizing both sugar and fat. Enjoy eggs for breakfast, and you'll be energizing your body and pumping up your muscle tone.

When it comes to convenience and ease of preparation, eggs really are the best protein money can buy, and because they provide more nutrients than calories, they earn the title "nutrient dense." Omega-3–enriched eggs, such as Eggland's Best, are available in most grocery stores across America. Why not add a dozen to your grocery list today?

Recommended Usage

Up to two eggs per day, preferably omega-3–enriched eggs.

Just the Facts

- There is no nutritional difference between white and brown eggs. However, if you make hard-boiled eggs frequently, select brown eggs. They have a thicker shell and won't crack as easily.
- Two omega-3–enriched eggs provide about half the recommended daily intake of omega-3 fatty acids.
- Eggs contain the highest quality of food protein known, second only to mother's milk.
- If you happen to drop an egg, cover it with salt and wait about 10 minutes. Cleanup will be a breeze!

Boost the Benefits

- When shopping for eggs, open the carton and make sure the eggs are clean and the shells aren't cracked.
- It's fine to buy organic, or free-range, eggs, but look for the words "omega-3–enriched" on the carton. Not all organic eggs are high in omega-3 fatty acids.
- Keep eggs refrigerated at all times, and they will maintain their freshness for several weeks. In fact, properly stored, eggs rarely spoil. If you keep them long enough, they are likely to simply dry up. However, at room temperature, eggs age more in one day than they do in one week in the refrigerator.
- Keep eggs in their original carton so that they do not lose moisture or pick up odors and flavors from other foods. Do not store them in the refrigerator door since repeated opening of the door exposes them to too much heat.
- Do not use an egg if it is cracked or leaking.
- After making hard-boiled eggs, store them in their shells in the original carton. Use them within one week. And if you notice a "gassy" odor in your refrigerator, remember that it is harmless and will disappear in a few hours. The smell comes from the hydrogen sulfide formed when eggs are hard-boiled.
- To freeze raw eggs, beat them until blended, pour them into a freezer container, seal it tightly, and freeze. But don't freeze hard-boiled eggs, because freezing will make them tough and watery.

THINK TWICE!

- *To eliminate concern about eggshells carrying bacteria, clean your eggs with a Clorox wash.*

* *Always wash your hands with warm, soapy water after contact with raw eggs.*

Be a Fat Flush Cook

* Hard-boiled eggs make a great snack and are easy to pack for on-the-go lunches.
* To cook eggs without added fat, try poaching them or use a nonstick pan with a bit of broth.
* For a healthy egg salad, chop some hard-boiled eggs and mix them with fresh lemon juice, flaxseed oil, minced onion, and dill.
* Serve a poached egg on a bed of steamed spinach for a vitamin-packed meal.
* Top scrambled eggs with homemade or organic salsa for a zesty breakfast.

Fat Flush Fun

* Take your eggs and place them in a bowl of water. A fresh egg will sink to the bottom and lie on its side, while an older egg will stand up on one end. If the egg is really old, it may even float.

IT'S BEEN SAID . . .

I've been eating two omega-3 enriched eggs per day for over 6 months. Recently, I had my cholesterol checked, and it was back to normal—for the first time in years. Both my LDL and HDL levels were great and my triglycerides were 91. Hurray!

BARBARA A., KENTUCKY

LAMB

Fat Flush Factors

Blood Sugar Stabilizer
Energizer

Sheep have been a source of food and wool for thousands of years and are currently the most abundant livestock in the world. Lamb is a dietary staple throughout the world, including the Middle East, New Zealand, and Australia. Yet throughout the United States, lamb has always taken a backseat to beef, pork, and veal. Statistics show that the average American consumes just over half a pound of lamb per year.

If you breeze by the lamb section every time you shop for groceries, you may want to reconsider. Lamb is lean and meaty and, unlike most red meats, is not "marbled" with saturated fat. Approximately 36 percent of the fat in lamb is saturated. The rest is monounsaturated or polyunsaturated—the "good" types of dietary fat.

Lamb boosts your immune system and encourages growth and healing by providing an ample amount of zinc. Zinc also helps maintain a steady blood sugar level and metabolic rate. Lamb energizes the body by supplying heme iron, a form of iron that is easily absorbed. On top of offering copper, manganese, selenium, and riboflavin, lamb is a good source of vitamin B12, which helps the body metabolize nutrients and prevents anemia by building red blood cells.

Recommended Usage

One or two servings of lamb per week.

Just the Facts

• Lamb is the meat from young sheep that are less than one year old.
• If you buy graded lamb, remember that the prime and choice cuts are the most tender and tasty but also have the higher fat content.
• Free-range lambs have a much finer texture and taste than those fed with grain.

Boost the Benefits

- When purchasing lamb, look for light-red, finely textured meat. The bones should be reddish and moist, and any fat should be white, not yellow.
- Store cuts of lamb in the coldest part of the refrigerator for up to three days. If you won't be using the meat within three days, pop it in the freezer, where chops and roasts will keep for six to nine months.
- Ground lamb should be refrigerated and used or frozen within 24 hours. You can keep ground lamb in the freezer for three to four months.

Be a Fat Flush Cook

- Make lamb kebabs by placing bite-sized pieces of lamb on a skewer, along with your favorite Fat Flush vegetables. Broil or grill and enjoy.
- Ground lamb makes delicious burgers. Season and cook as you would a hamburger.
- Braise lamb loin pieces in broth flavored with freshly minced garlic and a pinch of fennel.
- For a healthy twist on a traditional recipe, serve lamb with a mint yogurt sauce, which is made from plain yogurt, mint leaves, garlic, and cayenne.

SALMON

Fat Flush Factors
Blood Sugar Stabilizer
Cholesterol Zapper
Energizer

The salmon is an amazing creature, traveling thousands of miles throughout its life cycle and returning, within two to five years, to spawn and die at the very location where it was born. There are six species of salmon, five in the Pacific Ocean and just one in the Atlantic. Their flesh ranges in color from pink to red to orange, with some varieties containing more health-giving omega-3 fatty acids than others. For example, chinook and sockeye salmon are fattier fish than pink and chum and contain abundant amounts of omega-3s.

Salmon is hugely popular around the world. An average portion provides over half the daily recommended allowance of energy-promoting protein while dishing up less saturated fat than an equal portion of any meat or poultry. These delicious fish also contain carotenoids (yellow and orange pigments that serve as antioxidants), vitamins A and D, and several B vitamins. However, in nutrition circles, it is the polyunsaturated fatty acids for which salmon is best known. These "good" fats help reduce the risk of heart disease, lower cholesterol, and slow the onset of inflammatory diseases. In fact, one study found that women who ate salmon on a weekly basis were 30 percent less likely to die of heart disease than women who ate fish only once a month. Researchers have uncovered similar heart-healthy effects for men who eat fish regularly.

Remember, our bodies don't make essential fatty acids. It's up to us to provide them by eating the right kinds of foods. Studies have shown that about 60 percent of Americans are deficient in omega-3 essential fatty acids. So beef up your intake of omega-3s by putting salmon on your menu.

Recommended Usage

At least two servings of salmon per week.

Just the Facts

- Salmon is sold in many different forms. Fresh salmon comes whole or in steak or fillet form. You can also find frozen, canned, dried, or smoked salmon.
- Salmon may be wild or farm-raised. While both are rich in vitamins and essential fatty acids, you'll get the most nutritional value for your money with wild salmon.
- Norwegian salmon, a popular type of salmon often offered on restaurant menus, is actually Atlantic salmon that is farm-raised in Norway.

Boost the Benefits

- Fresh whole salmon should be displayed *buried* in ice, while fillets and steaks should be placed on top of the ice. Look for fish that is presented belly down so that the ice drains away from the fish as it melts. This reduces the chance of spoilage.
- If possible, smell salmon before buying it. Check for a mild "sea breeze" odor. If the fish smells like ammonia, it is definitely not fresh.
- Refrigerate salmon and prepare it within a day or two. Since most refrigerators are slightly warmer than ideal for storing fish, your best bet for maintaining freshness is to place salmon, tightly sealed in plastic wrap, in a baking dish filled with ice. Place the dish on the bottom shelf of the refrigerator and replenish the ice once or twice a day.
- You can prolong the shelf life of salmon by freezing it. Wrap it well in plastic and place it in the coldest part of the freezer, where it should keep for about two to three weeks.
- If you buy commercially frozen salmon, check the package for signs of thawing such as lumps and ice crystals.
- Use frozen fish within three months. To thaw frozen fish, defrost the fish in the refrigerator. Do not refreeze it.
- If purchasing canned salmon, make sure it is packed in water, not oil. To get rid of excess sodium, drain the fish in a strainer and then rinse it under cold water.

Be a Fat Flush Cook

- If you notice a foamy white substance on the surface of salmon as you cook it, you may have overcooked the fish or prepared it at too high a temperature. The "white stuff" is a harmless protein, but you may want to modify your cooking technique next time.
- In general, whether you bake, poach, broil, or grill your salmon, the cooking time for it is 10 minutes for every inch of thickness.

- To test for doneness, slip the point of a sharp knife into the thickest part of the fish and pull it aside. If flakes begin to separate, the fish is probably done and should be removed from the heat. Let it stand for three to four minutes to finish cooking.
- Use salmon in your favorite stir-fries, salads, soups, and even Mexican dishes, such as tacos or burritos.
- Broil or grill salmon steaks and sprinkle them with dried mustard and flaxseed oil.
- Spruce up plain fish with lemon or lime juice and herbs such as dill, garlic, or parsley.
- For a yummy change of pace, try making a salmon burger—made with canned salmon in place of ground beef. Shape the fish into a patty and brown it in a nonstick skillet.

THINK TWICE!

- *Government inspection is not mandated for seafood, so buy your salmon from a reputable fish counter or market.*
- *While some fish are not considered safe for pregnant or nursing mothers or young children to eat, eating wild Pacific salmon poses no safety concerns. At the seafood counter, ask for salmon marked as Alaskan salmon because it is guaranteed to be wild.*
- *Farm-raised salmon contains more contaminants than wild salmon because of overcrowding and exposure to feces.*

IT'S BEEN SAID . . .

When making salmon for dinner, I always grill an extra portion and save it to use as a topping for my lunch salad the next day. This saves time and helps keep me on track with my weight loss.

JANE V., IOWA

VEGAN PROTEINS: RICE AND PEA

Fat Flush Factors
Blood Sugar Stabilizer
Cholesterol Zapper
Energizer
Thermogenic

Getting plenty of protein in your daily diet is essential if you want to burn fat while building muscle, and protein powders can be very useful. Some claim that plant proteins are "more slimming" than dairy proteins such as whey, but the jury is still out as far as science is concerned. Dairy-derived proteins may lead to a bit more "bloat" for some individuals, although that's certainly not everyone's experience. I am a huge fan of whey protein, but I believe there is a place for both—so here's the scoop on vegan protein powders.

Some worry that plant proteins aren't as complete or effective as animal proteins when it comes to maintaining lean body mass; however, this is really a myth. All proteins are composed of amino acids, and as long as you're getting all nine of the essential amino acids that your body can't make for itself, then you're golden. Any protein containing all nine is considered a "complete protein."

A number of studies now indicate that plant-based diets result in better overall health, including lower rates of colon cancer and heart disease. Those people with compromised kidneys who consume more plant-based proteins have been found to accumulate fewer toxins in their blood than those who consume more animal proteins.

My favorite vegan proteins are derived from peas and rice—particularly a combination of the two. These proteins support weight loss, maintain lean body mass, sustain energy, and provide immune support and antiaging benefits. Pea protein is one of the most hypoallergenic proteins because it's free of dairy, gluten, peanuts, tree nuts, and soybeans—all of the most notorious allergens. Pea and rice proteins are also free of the phytoestrogens found in soy, and the vast majority of soybeans are genetically engineered, which is why I steer clear of soy-based protein powders.

Pea protein is also very satisfying. Studies have found that it rivals whey for staving off hunger pangs. Pea protein has been scientifically shown to lower levels of ghrelin, the "hunger hormone," due to an abundance of peptides that delay stomach emptying. Pea protein also has other health benefits, including lowering blood pressure and reducing your risk for heart disease and kidney disease. It's rich in soluble fiber, which is good for your lipid profile. And the cultivation of peas is environmentally friendly.

Although pea protein has a near-complete amino acid profile, it lacks a couple of nonessential amino acids (which your body produces). This is why I like combining pea protein with rice protein. Rice protein is a bit low in lysine—and pea protein nicely fills the gap.

High-quality rice proteins are usually extracted from sprouted brown rice and are very easy to digest, without spiking blood sugar. Rice protein is particularly beneficial after a workout because its leucine is rapidly absorbed. Leucine is an amino acid that slows muscle degradation. In a 2013 study, rice protein was found to be as beneficial as whey protein for body composition and exercise performance. Another study found brown rice protein to be more effective than white rice protein or soy protein for improving body composition and lipid profile. When it comes to your heart and liver, rice protein is the bomb—it optimizes cholesterol, reduces blood pressure, and protects your liver from oxidative damage. It may even offer some anticancer benefits. Two studies have shown that rice protein provides protection against breast cancer in rats and mice.

Regardless of the type of protein powders you choose, opt for organic, minimally processed whole-food protein concentrates, as opposed to overprocessed protein isolates that have had their cofactors stripped away, which compromises nutrient bioavailability.

Recommended Usage

- Consume one or two servings of vegan protein daily, depending on your activity level.
- A dose of vegan protein immediately after a workout may give you an edge. It's been established that the body can more readily absorb the amino acids in a protein shake for about 30 minutes after exertion, more efficiently than at any other time.

Boost the Benefits

- Combine or alternate between different protein powders to maximize benefits.
- Look for high-quality products made from whole-food sources, free of artificial sweeteners, gluten, dairy, egg, soy, etc. Watch for hidden sugars such as lactose, sugar, fructose, or crystalline fructose. Avoid any product sporting that long list of chemical ingredients that are impossible to pronounce.

- Look for a protein powder derived from sprouted brown rice, not simply "rice protein." Sprouting the rice reduces its carbohydrate content, increases protein, improves nutrient bioavailability, and lowers the overall glycemic effect.

Fat Flush in Action

- Mix protein powder into water or juice to make gangbuster smoothies. Add in a little coconut or MCT oil, flaxseed oil, macadamia nut oil, or tigernut oil to kick up the nutrition a few notches. How about a frozen smoothie for dessert?
- Protein powders can also be added to baked goods such as cookies and bars to bump up their nutritional value.
- Make a batter for crepe-like pancakes using protein powder, water, and eggs—and then top off with your favorite fruit.

THINK TWICE!

- *Many commercial protein powders—especially rice proteins—are contaminated with toxic lead, cadmium, mercury, arsenic, and tungsten. This is the last thing you want to be consuming during a detox! Whenever possible, go with brands that utilize third-party testing of their products for heavy-metal contamination.*

Fat Flush Fun

- In 2011, a group of health-conscious, enterprising firefighters began making cookies using a brown rice protein base in an effort to create healthier tasty treats for themselves and others in their New Jersey fire department. They have since founded "Cookie Republic," and to this day, they continue to produce delicious, nutritious brown rice cookies for the world to enjoy.

IT'S BEEN SAID . . .

Give peas a chance.

As you blend up your vegan smoothie, breathe deeply and "Visualize whirled peas."

ANONYMOUS

I like Rice. Rice is great if you're hungry and want two thousand of something.

MITCH HEDBERG

WHEY PROTEIN

Fat Flush Factors

Blood Sugar Stabilizer
Cholesterol Zapper
Energizer

Did you know that whey protein is the most easily absorbed, readily utilized protein, offering the most protein per serving? All that, and it's delicious, too! However, many people have never heard of whey protein, much less tasted it. Here's the scoop.

The two main proteins in milk are whey and casein. During the cheese-making process, these proteins are separated. The casein becomes cheese, and until recently, the whey was disposed of down the drain or treated as "slop" for farm animals. But not anymore. Now we know the value of this nutritionally complete protein. Unlike soy or wheat protein, whey contains all the essential amino acids and has the highest number of branched-chain amino acids, which are crucial for a strong and healthy body.

Research has shown that consumption of whey helps reduce the risk of breast and colon cancer, hypertension, and heart disease. It boosts the immune system by increasing the levels of glutathione, the most potent antioxidant in the body. Even dentists are pleased, since whey has been shown to reduce dental plaque and cavities.

In addition to increasing lean muscle mass and energizing the body, whey provides a number of other Fat Flush benefits. It helps keep blood sugar levels stable, which staves off the cravings that result from swings in your blood sugar. Components in whey help promote satiety by increasing the level of CCK, an appetite-suppressing hormone. Whey pumps up serotonin levels in the brain, which help fend off depression—and emotional eating.

The good news is that whey protein is easy and inexpensive to produce. But that's also the bad news. If you're not careful, you may end up with low-quality whey protein, which fails to produce the desired results. To maintain its integrity, whey protein must be processed under careful low-temperature and low-acid conditions.

To be considered a Fat Flush superfood, whey protein must be compliant with the strictest Fat Flush criteria; it must be lactose-free, have no added sugar, and contain no artificial sweeteners. The cow's milk used to produce the whey concentrate for the whey protein powder should be the highly sought-after nonmutated A2 beta-casein (milk protein). A1 beta-casein, found in most cow's milk from North America, may be linked to digestive problems, cardiovascular concerns, and diabetes. In addition to being easier to digest, A2 protein also contains the amino acid proline—which fights aging by supporting collagen. The only permissible sweetener is stevia or monk fruit with inulin, a substance that nourishes the GI tract with friendly bacteria.

Recommended Usage

One or two servings of whey protein daily (depending on your activity level).

Just the Facts

• Whey's historical use as a medicinal food goes as far back as 400 BC, to the time of Hippocrates.
• Because whey is so easily digested, it is a common ingredient in infant formulas and medically prescribed protein supplements.
• As the protein level of a whey protein increases, the amount of lactose it contains decreases.

Boost the Benefits

• Read the label carefully when buying whey protein. Whey protein *isolate* is the purest form of whey protein, containing between 90 and 95 percent protein and little to no fat or lactose. Whey protein *concentrate* is available in a number of different types based upon protein content, which can range from 25 to 89 percent.
• Be leery of buying whey protein out of a bulk bin. Inexpensive whey may be very low in protein and high in lactose. It may also have been cheaply processed at high temperatures, which reduces its nutritional value.
• Watch out, too, for hidden sugars or artificial sweeteners. Don't waste your money on whey protein that contains lactose, sugar, crystalline fructose, or artificial sweeteners such as aspartame, neotame, acesulfame K, sucralose, or Splenda. Do purchase whey protein that lists Stevia Plus or stevia with inulin, a natural herbal product, as its only sweetener.

Be a Fat Flush Cook

• Whey protein can be mixed with water or juice to make a pleasant-tasting and nutritious snack.

- Mix whey protein with your favorite frozen fruit and some cranberry juice. Add a dash of cinnamon, and you've got a terrific fat-burning meal or snack.
- Dissolve a bit of whey protein in water to make a substitute for cream in your herbal or organic coffee.
- Combine whey protein, water, and eggs to make a batter for crepe-like pancakes. Top them with your favorite fruit.

THINK TWICE!

- *Many people who have experienced lactose intolerance have no trouble consuming whey protein, especially if they select a pure whey protein isolate.*

IT'S BEEN SAID . . .

What would I do without my whey protein smoothies? I used to skip breakfast, but now I have a Fat Flush whey smoothie every morning. It keeps me satisfied for hours, and I've dropped ten pounds in three weeks!

BECKY Z., CALIFORNIA

3 Fat Flush Vegetables

When diet is wrong, medicine is of no use.
When diet is correct, medicine is of no need.

—ANCIENT AYURVEDIC PROVERB

Vegetables in all hues and shades are loaded with healing phytonutrients and antioxidants to revitalize health. Little did we know that when our mothers told us to "eat our vegetables," it was some of the best advice we'd receive in our entire lives. Study after study has confirmed that people who eat more vegetables than other folks have a lower risk of developing chronic diseases and stand a good chance of maintaining a high quality of life well into their senior years.

From asparagus to zucchini, vegetables offer us a wealth of vitamins, fiber, and minerals, all of which are necessary for our well-being. Because our bodies can't stockpile these nutrients, we need to eat a variety of vegetables every day to ensure optimal health. A recent study by the National Cancer Institute found that Americans are indeed eating more vegetables than they did 25 years ago. Sadly, at least one-fourth of those additional vegetables are french fries.

Obviously, you won't find fried potatoes among the Fat Flush vegetables in this chapter. However, you will find a delicious assortment of Mother Nature's bounty—vegetables that will help you maintain a healthy weight, reduce your risk of heart disease and diabetes, and offer protection against cancer. By decorating your dinner plate with a rainbow of vegetables (like leafy greens, squash, beets, and purple produce), you'll fortify your body with the colorful pigments that give vegetables their antioxidant, disease-fighting power. In total, plant foods contain over 5,000 antioxidants, including anthocyanins in purple green beans and eggplants, sulforaphane in broccoli, flavonoids in cabbages, and lycopene in tomatoes, all of which are potent anti-inflammatories, help protect the heart, and stave off aging.

The 12 vegetables discussed in this chapter were chosen because they are Fat Flush superfoods and provide a healthy balance of green, orange, and red or purple "pigment power." If you mix and match these nutritious plant foods and eat generous daily portions as detailed in the New Fat

Flush Plan, you'll begin to notice a number of exciting side effects. Water retention will be a thing of the past, your cellulite will start to disappear, your skin will take on a healthy glow, and those snug clothes in your closet will suddenly fit like a glove. Better still, your blood tests will make you and your doctor smile!

ASPARAGUS

Fat Flush Factors
Detoxifier
Diuretic

First cultivated in Greece about 2,500 years ago, asparagus offers a delicate, Fat Flush flavor and tender texture. Originally, asparagus was used by the ancient Greeks and Romans to relieve toothaches and prevent bee stings, but today it is well known as a diuretic. This vegetable's ability to fight water retention comes from the fact that it is high in potassium and low in sodium and contains an amino acid called asparagine. This trio also helps prevent fatigue by neutralizing ammonia, a substance that can build up in our bodies during the digestive process.

While asparagus may be considered a luxury vegetable, it pays for itself in nutritional benefits. Asparagus contains a special carbohydrate called inulin that is not digested but helps feed the friendly bacteria in the large intestine. When we consume inulin regularly, these friendly bacteria proliferate, keeping the intestinal tract clear of unfriendly bacteria. In addition, asparagus is an excellent source of glutathione, an important anticarcinogen, and rutin, a substance that protects small blood vessels from rupturing.

There's more good news. Asparagus provides vitamins A and C, potassium, phosphorus, and iron. It's also a good source of fiber, the B-complex vitamins, and zinc. These delicate spears are also high in folic acid, which has been shown to reduce the risk of heart disease. Researchers believe that consuming 400 micrograms of folic acid per day would decrease the heart attack rate in the United States by 10 percent. Just one serving of asparagus provides over half of this recommended amount.

Recommended Usage
At least a half-cup to one-cup serving of asparagus per week.

Just the Facts
* Asparagus is a member of the lily family. While there are approximately 300 varieties of asparagus, only 20 of them are edible.

- Female asparagus stalks are plumper than male stalks and can grow as much as 10 inches in one day.
- The color of an asparagus spear, not its thickness, determines how tender it will be. Deep green or pure white spears are usually the most tender.
- White asparagus is not a different variety from the traditional green; it is simply grown in darkness. Green asparagus has a higher vitamin content than the white.

Boost the Benefits

- When you're shopping, look for straight asparagus stalks with firm stems of equal thickness. The tips should be tight, come to a point, and be deep green or purplish in color. Partially open or wilted tips are a hint that the asparagus is past its prime. Avoid asparagus that is excessively dirty or sandy.
- To ensure freshness, select asparagus that has been kept refrigerated or displayed upright in trays of cold water.
- The size of the stalk is not a measure of quality, but rather personal preference. While asparagus is usually found in bundles, you may see it sold loose. If so, select spears of the same size to ensure even cooking.
- To prevent rapid spoiling, always unband asparagus spears before storing them. Wrap the ends in a damp paper towel, place the spears in a plastic bag, and store the asparagus in your refrigerator.
- Since folate is destroyed by exposure to light, make a place in the *back* of the refrigerator for asparagus.
- While asparagus will keep for four or five days in the refrigerator, its flavor will diminish with each passing day. It's best to prepare and eat it the day you buy it.

Be a Fat Flush Cook

- When you're planning your menu, keep in mind that trimming and cooking causes asparagus to lose about half its total weight. A pound of asparagus serves two people as a main dish; three or four people as a side dish.
- Before cooking, snap off the tough bottom end of each asparagus stalk. But don't throw away those ends. Peel them and toss them in a pot of soup.
- You can buy a special asparagus steamer that holds the stalks upright while they cook. However, you may use any tall, lidded pot or a collapsible vegetable steamer placed in a large skillet.

- Cook asparagus *quickly*, or it becomes limp and discolored and takes on a bitter taste. Five to ten minutes should do the trick. To test for doneness, try to pierce the bottom of a stalk with the end of a paring knife. If the knife goes in, the asparagus is ready.
- For a different twist, add a clove of garlic, a slice of onion, or a lemon wedge to the water when you're cooking asparagus.
- After cooking, let the asparagus spears drain on a paper towel for a minute before serving. If you plan to serve the asparagus cold, rinse it with cold water right away to stop the cooking process.
- Are you tired of plain scrambled eggs? Add a bit of chopped asparagus to give them color and flavor.

THINK TWICE!

- Cooking asparagus in a metal pan can cause discoloration of the metal.
- If you notice a strong odor to your urine after eating asparagus, don't panic. The harmless odor is caused by a chemical called methyl mercaptan, a by-product of the breakdown of asparagus.

IT'S BEEN SAID . . .

I marinate a pound of asparagus in ¼ cup flax oil, 1 clove crushed garlic, 1 tsp fresh minced onion, 3 tbsp lemon juice, and a dash of cayenne. After letting it stand for one hour, the asparagus is ready to eat or to chop and add to a tossed salad.

DEBRA F., CALIFORNIA

BEETS

Fat Flush Factors
Blood Sugar Stabilizer
Cholesterol Zapper
Detoxifier

Beets are one of the most regenerative foods for your body. It's hard to keep up with their ever-expanding list of benefits, which seems to grow longer by the day. Beets aid digestion, thin the bile, cleanse the liver, alkalize the blood, and even improve cognitive function and sports performance. The Green Med Info database lists beets' therapeutic actions as antihypertensive, lipid-lowering, detoxifying, anti-inflammatory, antioxidant, antibacterial, hepatoprotective, neuroprotective, and anticancer—which is quite the résumé for one food group.

Beets are rich in potassium, manganese, copper, magnesium, phosphorous, vitamin C, iron, folate, vitamin B6, nitrates, and fiber—among others. Their carotenoid pigments (betalains) have a number of benefits as well. Beet greens and yellow beetroots are rich in lutein and zeaxanthin, which benefit your eyes and nervous system. The betalains partner with glutathione to help your body detox. The fiber in beets helps prevent constipation, and their nitrates boost endurance. Just one single dose of beet juice has been shown to improve cognitive function.

If you're concerned about weight loss, beets are your best friend because of their benefits for your liver and gallbladder. First, beets are rich in betaine, which thins the bile and helps prevent gallstones. Betaine is a derivative of choline and is found in the peel and fleshy part of the beet. Betaine is also a rich source of hydrochloric acid and triggers the release of bile by your gallbladder—which, it is hoped, you still possess. Betaine is known for its ability to reduce homocysteine levels by conversion to methionine. Homocysteine is a toxic amino acid that increases your risk for cardiovascular disease and osteoporosis. Betaine also increases serotonin, which can boost mood.

Beets help build strong bile. What does bile have to do with losing weight? Bile is responsible for breaking down fats so they can be used for fuel, instead of padding for your hips and thighs. And bile requires the assistance of your gallbladder.

The gallbladder is a muscular pear-shaped organ next to your liver. Your liver produces about 1 to 1½ quarts of bile per day, which it makes from cholesterol. Your liver sends bile to your gallbladder for storage and concentration. Adding bile to the food in your gut is like adding soap to your dishwater—it breaks down and disperses the fat. When fats pass from your stomach into your intestine, your gallbladder receives a message to release bile in order to emulsify the fats, which prepares them for further processing by the pancreatic enzyme lipase. Once bile is used up, your liver must produce more of it, and it uses cholesterol for this. Therefore, beets help optimize cholesterol levels.

When bile is insufficient or too thick and "sludgy," oversized fat globules make their way into your bloodstream. Because they're not properly broken down, your body can't use them for fuel, so it stores them in fat cells instead . . . helloooo cellulite. Bile is also a powerful antioxidant that helps detoxify your liver.

Bile acids have multiple functions such as increasing the metabolic activity of brown fat, flushing little gallstones out of the liver, improving insulin sensitivity, stimulating the production of active thyroid hormone in fat cells, and helping your body absorb calcium, iron, and fat-soluble vitamins A, D, E, and K. The latest research shows that bile acids also trigger regeneration in damaged areas of the liver.

Beets are not a substitute for bile acids, but their betaine does stimulate and protect your liver and bile ducts.

If you've had your gallbladder removed, building up your bile is even *more* important. Gallbladder removal is one of the most common surgeries in the United States today. Without a gallbladder to store bile, the bile continuously trickles into your intestine regardless of whether you've consumed fat. Then, when you do consume a fatty meal, there is no reserve, and over time this can result in packing on the pounds, as well as developing nutritional deficiencies.

The last way beets can help you is by acting as a bile sequestrant. A significant portion of spent bile acids is reabsorbed by your body, from your intestine back into your bloodstream, along with the toxins bound to them. Beets come to the rescue! Many vegetables are natural "bile sequestrants," meaning they bind to bile acids in your intestine and prevent their reabsorption so they can be eliminated via your stool. A USDA study compared the bile-binding potential of various veggies—cabbage, cauliflower, mustard greens, broccoli, kale, and several others—and beets topped the list.

Recommended Usage

- Beets are delicious juiced or grated raw onto salads.
- Beet greens are delicious sautéed like spinach—and like spinach, they wilt down quickly, so be careful to not overcook them.

- Beets lend themselves well to pickling. Try beets pickled in apple cider vinegar and paired with hard-boiled eggs for a healthy snack.
- What about a shredded beet slaw with citrus dressing? Beets and oranges are a match made in heaven.
- Try simmering beets and tomatoes in stock, and puree for a colorful, antioxidant-rich winter soup. Or make "borscht," a classic European beet soup with dozens of variations.
- Puree beets into hummus for added color and nutrition.
- Beet puree added to "red velvet" chocolate cake creates a more nutritious (and moister) dessert.

Just the Facts

- Traditionally, beets were used as a folk remedy for liver disorders.
- Beet greens and stalks were originally consumed like chard. Then around 1542, the root part of the beet was cultivated in either Germany or Italy. Early beetroots were shaped more like parsnips than the bulbous forms seen today.
- Because beets and beet juice are alkaline, they help alkalize your blood.

Boost the Benefits

- Beet leaves last only a few days in your fridge, but the roots can stay fresh for two or three weeks. It's best to store them separately.
- Steaming beetroot significantly improves its bile acid–binding capacity.

Fat Flush in Action

- Beet kvass is a beverage made by fermenting beets in water. Kvass has all the benefits of beets with none of the sugar—plus the added benefit of lactic acid bacteria. Sally Fallon's famous *Nourishing Traditions* cookbook has an easy recipe for beet kvass, and all you need are a few beetroots, sea salt, water, and a little natural whey or sauerkraut juice to kick off the fermentation process.

Be a Fat Flush Cook

- Beets rapidly lose their pigments when cooked. The red betalains in beets are far less heat stable than red anthocyanin pigments in red cabbage. In order to preserve these beneficial pigments, cut beets into quarters (with the skin intact) and steam them for no more than 15 minutes, or roast them for up to 1 hour.

THINK TWICE!

- Beets may turn your urine (beeturia) and stool a reddish color.
- They are high in oxalate, so you might want to avoid them if you are prone to kidney stones or gout.
- If you suffer from hemochromatosis, be careful not to overconsume beet juice, as it may lead to an overaccumulation of metals such as iron, copper, magnesium, and phosphorous.

Fat Flush Fun

- Beet juice is being investigated as an aid for altitude sickness. The nitrates in beets convert to nitric oxide, which relaxes blood vessels and makes it easier for your body to function in low-oxygen conditions.

IT'S BEEN SAID . . .

Visitors to Russia can observe the following typical sight on Moscow street corners: a large metal drum, larger than a beer keg, turned sideways and mounted on wheels. A spigot on one end releases a brown bubbly liquid into a glass. Customers line up to pay for a draught, down it in several gulps and return the glass to the vendor who wipes it clean for the next customer. . . . Kvass can also be made from beets. The result is not so much epicurean as medicinal, although beet kvass is often added to borscht.

SALLY FALLON MORELL

Some historians say that beets were offered to the goddess Aphrodite to maintain and enhance her beauty.

BROCCOLI

Fat Flush Factors

Blood Sugar Stabilizer
Cholesterol Zapper
Detoxifier

A close relative of cauliflower, broccoli has been part of the American diet for over 200 years. Yet it wasn't until a 1930s radio campaign championing the benefits of broccoli that the public really caught on to this highly nutritious vegetable. Not only does broccoli provide a variety of textures, from soft to crunchy, but it also hits the jackpot as a Fat Flush food. Iron, vitamin C, potassium, fiber—broccoli has all these and more! Munching on broccoli gives you abundant amounts of folic acid, calcium, and vitamin A.

Like other cruciferous vegetables, broccoli gives a boost to certain enzymes that help detoxify the body. Detoxification contributes to weight loss while helping to prevent cancer, diabetes, heart disease, osteoporosis, and high blood pressure. Worried about your cholesterol? Broccoli is known to contain a certain *pectin fiber* that binds to bile acids and keeps cholesterol from being released into the bloodstream. Does diabetes run in your family? At the USDA's Human Research Laboratory, a diabetes expert found that the chromium in broccoli may be effective in preventing type 2 diabetes by maintaining stable blood sugar levels.

In other research, at Johns Hopkins University, sulforaphane, a chemical found in broccoli, was found to kill *H. pylori*, bacteria that cause stomach ulcers and stomach cancers. Sulforaphane even destroyed those strains of the bacteria that had become resistant to antibiotics. Broccoli is also a good source of folic acid, which scientists now believe serves as a defense against Alzheimer's disease. In addition, broccoli has been singled out as one of the few vegetables that significantly reduce the risk of heart disease.

How's that for a deal? For just pennies per serving, broccoli serves up a feast of fat-flushing properties and helps keep you lean, strong, and healthy!

Recommended Usage

At least three to five cups of broccoli per week.

Just the Facts

- The word *broccoli* comes from the Latin word *brachium*, which means "strong arm" or "branch."
- Some broccoli hybrids include broccolini, a cross between broccoli and Chinese kale; broccoflower, a cross between broccoli and cauliflower; and purple broccoli, a cousin of broccoli, which looks like small heads of purple cauliflower.
- Ounce for ounce, broccoli offers more vitamin C than an orange and as much calcium as a glass of milk. One medium spear has three times more fiber than a slice of wheat bran bread and over 1,000 IUs of vitamin A.
- Broccoli sprouts are tiny three-day-old plants that resemble alfalfa sprouts and have a peppery flavor. Researchers estimate that, depending on their age, broccoli sprouts contain up to 100 times the nutritional power of mature broccoli.
- A typical bunch of broccoli weighs about two pounds, which is enough to serve as a side dish for three or four people.

Boost the Benefits

- You can rely on the color of broccoli to serve as an indicator of its nutritional value. Florets that are dark green, purplish, or bluish green contain more beta-carotene and vitamin C than paler florets. Select broccoli with compact floret clusters that are uniform in color.
- Bypass broccoli that is bruised or yellowed or that has a brown or slimy stalk. And if you see yellow flowers beginning to blossom within the clusters, the broccoli is overripe and will be tough and woody—no matter how you cook it.
  Fresh broccoli has a clean "green" smell, so if you notice a strong odor, the broccoli is past its prime.
- Fresh broccoli is at its best if it is used within a day or two of purchase, but it will keep for up to four days if stored in your refrigerator's crisper. Alternatively, you can stand broccoli up, bouquet style, in a jar of water, cover it with a plastic bag, and store it on a shelf in the fridge.
- If you have an abundance of broccoli, don't let it go bad. Instead, blanch it and then pop it in the freezer where it will keep for up to one year.

Be a Fat Flush Cook

- Very fresh, young broccoli is tender enough to be served raw or tossed in a salad.

- Do you throw away broccoli leaves? If so, you're discarding the highest concentration of beta-carotene. The leaves are edible, so try adding them to your salad greens.
- Cooked broccoli should be tender enough so that you can pierce the stalks with a sharp knife, but it should still be crisp and bright. To ensure that the stalks cook as quickly as the florets, cut an X in the bottom of each stalk and/or a lengthwise slit in the stems.
- Sprinkle lemon juice and ground flax seeds over lightly steamed broccoli.
- Chop some broccoli and add it to your morning omelet.

THINK TWICE!

- *Like its cruciferous relatives, broccoli contains goitrogens, naturally occurring substances that can interfere with thyroid function. If you have been diagnosed with a thyroid disorder, you may want to check with your physician before you consume large amounts of broccoli.*
- *Keep in mind that packaged, frozen broccoli contains twice as much sodium and fewer health-promoting phytochemicals compared to fresh broccoli.*

Fat Flush Fun

- Do not let the smell of the sulfur compounds released while broccoli is cooking keep you away from this nutritious vegetable. Drop a large piece of stale bread in the cooking water to counteract the odor.

IT'S BEEN SAID . . .

I have found that the Fat Flush herbs and spices that go best with broccoli include dill, mustard seed, cayenne, and garlic.

DIANE L., NEW YORK

I do not like broccoli. And I haven't liked it since I was a little kid and my mother made me eat it. And I'm President of the United States and I'm not going to eat any more broccoli.

GEORGE BUSH, U.S. PRESIDENT, 1990

CABBAGE

Fat Flush Factors
Detoxifier

One of the world's oldest vegetables, cabbage continues to be an inexpensive dietary staple. Because it is easy to grow, we are lucky enough to find this nutritional powerhouse throughout the year, although it is at its best during the late fall and winter.

A member of the cruciferous family, which includes broccoli and kale, cabbage is rich in cancer-fighting nutrients, including vitamin C, fiber, and two phytochemicals, sulforaphane and indoles. These two compounds help detoxify the body, ridding it of cancer-producing substances, including excess estrogen. A number of studies have shown that women who include cabbage regularly in their diet reduce their risk of breast cancer by 45 percent.

Cabbage has powerful antibacterial properties as well. Decades ago, researchers at Stanford University determined that consuming cabbage is a good treatment for peptic ulcers. Glutamine is an amino acid that nourishes the cells that line the stomach and small intestine. The high glutamine content of cabbage allows it to heal ulcers, often in as few as 10 days. So if your consumption of cabbage has been limited to coleslaw or sauerkraut, take another look at this fantastic Fat Flush vegetable.

Recommended Usage
At least three ½-cup to 1-cup servings of cabbage per week.

Just the Facts
- At least a hundred different types of cabbage are grown throughout the world, but the most common types in the United States are the green, red, and Savoy varieties. Both green and red cabbages have smooth-textured leaves, while Savoy leaves are ruffled.
- The outer cabbage leaves are darker and contain more nutrients than the pale inner leaves, which develop without the benefit of sunlight.

Boost the Benefits

- Buy solid, heavy cabbage heads with shiny, crisp, colorful leaves. Watch out for cracks, bruises, and blemishes because damage to the outer leaves suggests hidden worm damage or decay.
- If there are no outer leaves on the cabbage, it means that the head has already been trimmed and may well have come from storage rather than from a fresh harvest.
- Once cabbage is cut, it loses its vitamin C content rapidly. So while buying precut cabbage may be convenient, it will cost you important nutrients.
- Keeping cabbage cold keeps it fresh and helps retain its vitamin C content. Place the whole head in a perforated plastic bag in the crisper of your refrigerator, where it will stay fresh for about two weeks.
- Once the head has been cut, place the remainder in a plastic bag in the refrigerator. Your best bet is to use it up in a day or two.
- Because phytonutrients in the cabbage react with carbon steel, turning the leaves black, cut it with a stainless-steel knife.

Be a Fat Flush Cook

- Cut up fresh cabbage and sprinkle it with lemon, and you've got a delicious afternoon snack.
- Throw in some chopped cabbage when making vegetable soup.
- Toss shredded red and white cabbage with fresh lemon juice and a bit of flaxseed or olive oil. Spice it up with some turmeric, cumin, coriander, and cayenne to make colorful coleslaw with a Fat Flush twist.
- Use cabbage leaves as a wrapper for cooked meats or veggies.
- Steam some sliced cabbage and top it with your favorite spaghetti sauce.
- Top a chicken sandwich with some shredded cabbage.

IT'S BEEN SAID . . .

For a filling Fat Flush side dish, I like to combine some red cabbage with a chopped apple. I simmer it in some salt-free vegetable broth, and it's ready to serve in minutes!

WENDY W., OREGON

The cabbage surpasses all other vegetables. If, at a banquet, you wish to dine a lot and enjoy your dinner, then eat as much cabbage as you wish, seasoned with vinegar, before dinner, and likewise after dinner eat some half-dozen leaves. It will make you feel as if you had not eaten, and you can drink as much as you like.

MARCUS PORCIUS CATO (ROMAN POLITICIAN, 234–149 BC)

CAULIFLOWER

Fat Flush Factors
Detoxifier

This is one versatile veggie, now known as "the new kale." You will find it taking center stage in cauliflower rice, as a potato substitute in mashed cauliflower, and as a creative pizza crust these days. Originating in ancient Asia, cauliflower is in the same cruciferous family as broccoli, kale, cabbage, and collards. However, because its heavy green leaves shield the flowering head from the sun, cauliflower lacks the green chlorophyll found in its "cousins." Instead, it remains milky white, with a spongy texture and sweet, slightly nutty flavor.

Cauliflower contains a high amount of vitamin C, folate, fiber, and complex carbohydrates. As a cruciferous vegetable, cauliflower has been studied for its role in reducing the risk of cancer. Scientists know that, for people with cancer, it is essential to rapidly detoxify toxins in the liver before they have a chance to encourage cell deregulation and uncontrolled cancerous growth. Cauliflower contains both glucosinolates and thiocyanates, compounds that increase the liver's ability to neutralize potential toxins. There are a number of enzymes in cauliflower, such as glutathione transferase, that also help with the detoxifying process.

Detoxification is also essential to weight loss and general health, so give cauliflower a prominent spot on your Fat Flush menu.

Recommended Usage

At least three cups of cauliflower per week.

Just the Facts

- The compact head of a cauliflower is called a "curd" and is composed of undeveloped flower buds.
- A medium-sized cauliflower head, measuring six inches in diameter and weighing about two pounds, will serve four people.

Boost the Benefits

• When shopping for cauliflower, look for creamy white heads that are firm, compact, and heavy for their size. Just say no to cauliflower with brown patches or spots.

• You'll get a fresher head of cauliflower if it is protected by a number of thick leaves.

• Should you pick a small or a large cauliflower? Size does not affect taste or quality, so go with the one that suits your needs.

• Buying precut cauliflower florets is probably not the best choice because they will lose their freshness after a day or two.

• If refrigerated in a perforated plastic bag, uncooked cauliflower will keep for up to a week. To prevent moisture from settling in the floret clusters, store the head with the leaves still on and the stem side down.

• Cooked cauliflower spoils faster, so don't store it in the refrigerator longer than a day or two.

Be a Fat Flush Cook

• Experiment with cauliflower rice or cauliflower mashed potatoes. Flavor with dill, garlic, and olive oil, and you'll never miss the real McCoy.

• When heated, cauliflower releases a sulfur-like odor that some people find unpleasant. The longer you cook cauliflower, the stronger the odor. So to minimize the smell—and preserve the nutrients—cook cauliflower for only a short time.

• Cauliflower may turn yellow if it is prepared in alkaline water. For whiter cauliflower, add a tablespoon or two of lemon juice to the cooking water.

• Don't waste those cauliflower stems and leaves. They are terrific for adding to soup stocks.

• For creating cauliflower with a surprising yellow color, boil it briefly with a spoonful of turmeric.

• Simmer cauliflower florets in a bit of broth with freshly minced garlic and ginger.

• For a quick soup, puree cooked cauliflower and add fennel seeds and your other favorite Fat Flush herbs and spices. Serve hot or cold.

• Don't forget that raw cauliflower makes a great, portable snack. It also adds texture and taste to your favorite tossed salad.

• Add chopped cauliflower florets to your favorite pasta sauce.

THINK TWICE!

- If you have been diagnosed with a thyroid condition, you may want to stick to cooked cauliflower. Cooking inactivates the goitrogenic compounds found in cauliflower. These substances occur naturally in certain foods and can interfere with thyroid function.
- Do not cook cauliflower in an aluminum or iron pot. Aluminum reacts with the phytochemicals in cauliflower and causes the florets to turn yellow, while iron causes cauliflower to take on a brownish or blue-green hue.

IT'S BEEN SAID . . .

I've never left the table hungry when mashed cauliflower is part of my meal. And it's so easy to prepare! Just steam some cauliflower, mash with a bit of broth and your favorite herbs . . . and voilà! You've got a terrific Fat Flush substitute for mashed potatoes.

KARI W., ILLINOIS

Cauliflower is nothing but cabbage with a college education.

MARK TWAIN

CUCUMBERS

Fat Flush Factors
Diuretic

Originating in Asia over 10,000 years ago, cucumbers are grown for slicing or pickling. Slicing, or "table," cucumbers are cylindrical in shape and usually range in length from six to nine inches, while pickling "cukes" are smaller. If you see a foot-long cucumber, it is probably an English or hothouse variety.

The pale-green flesh of a cucumber is mostly water, making it a moist and cooling treat. This fresh-tasting veggie adds crunch and fiber to any meal, while offering plenty of vitamin C, silica, potassium, and magnesium. A cucumber's vitamin C content helps calm irritated skin and reduce swelling, which is why cucumber slices are placed on eyelids at expensive spas to soothe tired, puffy eyes.

However, cucumbers do more than restore the sparkle to your eyes. Since silica is an essential component of healthy connective tissue, cucumbers help build strong muscles, tendons, and bones. Studies have shown that the minerals in cucumbers can fight hypertension by reducing systolic blood pressure by at least five points. And a generous helping of fat-flushing cucumber works to hydrate the body and reduce excess water weight.

Recommended Usage
One cucumber daily.

Just the Facts
- Because a cucumber is 95 percent water, its inside can be up to 20 degrees cooler than its outside temperature.
- Technically, the cucumber is a fruit and is related to the watermelon.
- Columbus brought the first cucumber seed to America.
- While cucumber seeds are edible, some people find the seedless English cucumber easier to digest.

Boost the Benefits

- Look for cucumbers with smooth, bright skin and an even green color. They should be firm, with no withered or shriveled ends.
- Steer clear of cucumbers that are yellow or that have sunken areas.
- Size does matter! In general, smaller cucumbers have a sweeter taste and fewer seeds than larger cucumbers.
- If you refrigerate cucumbers quickly after purchase, they should keep for about one week. However, since they are sensitive to temperature extremes, place your cucumbers close to the top of the fridge, which is often warmer. Storing them in a paper or cloth bag will keep them from catching a "chill."
- Most cucumbers are waxed to protect them from bruising during shipping. If you buy waxed cucumbers, be sure to peel them before you eat them. You'll save time, nutrients, *and* color by selecting unwaxed cucumbers, which may be eaten with the skin on. Organic cucumbers are a good choice, as are English cucumbers, which are wrapped in plastic.
- If cucumbers are exposed to weather extremes as they grow, they can develop a bitter taste. If you come across a bitter cucumber, discard an inch or so from the stem end, remove the seeds, and peel the entire cucumber. This should get rid of most of the harsh flavor.
- To seed a cucumber, peel it and cut it in half lengthwise. With the tip of a spoon or a melon baller, scrape the center from top to bottom to scoop out the seeds from each half.

Be a Fat Flush Cook

- Serving suggestion: Often, cucumbers straight out of the fridge are too cold to eat comfortably. Consider taking them out of the fridge when you first begin your meal preparation.
- Are you looking for a quick and easy snack? Slice a cucumber and enjoy it raw.
- Add sliced cucumber to your tossed salads.
- When you are making a sandwich, forget the second piece of bread. Top your sandwiches with crispy cucumber slices instead. Cook sliced cucumbers with your favorite Fat Flush herbs.
- For a tasty side dish, combine cucumber slices with thinly sliced red onion, plain yogurt, and fresh dill.
- Add diced cucumber to tuna fish or chicken salad recipes.

THINK TWICE!

- Cucumbers can cause an unpleasant mouth itch in people who are allergic to pollen or aspirin.
- The wax used on cucumbers may be a plant, insect, animal, or petroleum-based product. To avoid problems with these "unknown" substances, choose organic cucumbers.

IT'S BEEN SAID . . .

One of my favorite salads is a mixture of diced cucumbers with snow peas, tossed with some flax oil and apple cider vinegar. I add some fresh parsley and a dash of cayenne.

VICKY S., TEXAS

JICAMA

Fat Flush Factors
Cholesterol Zapper

Like many other Fat Flushers, I find jicama to be a cross between a potato and an apple—with a bit of water chestnut thrown in for good measure. This large, bulbous root is a popular Mexican vegetable with a sweet flavor and crunchy texture. Because jicama can be used either raw or cooked, it is a very versatile vegetable. Even cooked, it retains its crisp, water chestnut type of texture and flavor.

With its increasing popularity across the United States, more and more supermarkets are carrying jicama. Look for a brownish-gray root vegetable, shaped something like a turnip—or ask the produce manager to point you in the right direction. Extremely nutritious, jicama is low in sodium and contains no fat, making it a dieter's delight. A cup of jicama provides nearly six grams of fiber, which helps to satisfy the appetite and aid the digestive process. In addition, jicama is bursting with vitamin C. One of vitamin C's important functions is to keep LDL cholesterol from oxidizing—for only cholesterol that has been damaged by oxidation causes heart disease. Vitamin C may also protect against heart disease by "relaxing" stiff arteries and preventing platelets from clumping together.

As jicama becomes better known throughout kitchens in the United States, it will continue to show up in salads and stir-fries everywhere. If you haven't yet tried this unusual vegetable, give it a whirl. No doubt, you will enjoy it as much as I do.

Recommended Usage
One cup daily or as desired.

Just the Facts
- You may hear jicama called a yam bean, Mexican potato, or Chinese turnip.
- Jicama is pronounced "HEE-kuh-muh."
- Raw jicama tastes something like a nice crisp apple or pear.
- "Arrowroot," a common cooking thickener, is made from jicama.

Boost the Benefits

- At the store, look for a firm, heavy jicama that has smooth, relatively unblemished skin.
- While jicama can weigh up to six pounds, the smaller roots, weighing three pounds or less, offer better flavor and more juice than the larger ones.
- Store a whole jicama in a cool, dry place, because too much moisture can cause mold. It should stay fresh for up to two weeks.
- To avoid discoloration of the flesh, wash and peel jicama just before using it.
- Once you cut into the jicama, wrap any cut pieces in plastic and refrigerate them. They should maintain their freshness and flavor for one week.

Be a Fat Flush Cook

- Sliced or grated jicama adds a crunchy texture to any salad or slaw.
- For a delicious snack, try cutting jicama into cubes and mixing them with lime juice and a dusting of cayenne.
- Jicama may also be baked, boiled, or mashed like potatoes.
- When jicama is combined with other foods, it tends to take on the flavors of those ingredients. This ability to blend with other vegetables and seasonings makes jicama a lovely complement to stir-fry dishes.
- If you substitute jicama for water chestnuts in any recipe, you'll save some pennies!

IT'S BEEN SAID . . .

I've dropped fifteen pounds in two months of fat flushing, and jicama has really helped. I eat it every day as an afternoon snack. Sometimes I eat it plain; other times I spice it up with cayenne or cinnamon. It satisfies my urge to crunch . . . and has taken the place of potato chips in my life!

MARY F., KANSAS

KALE

One of the top vegetable sources of vitamin A, kale is a leafy green vegetable that belongs to the same family as cabbage, collards, and brussels sprouts. In fact, kale is known as the "grandmother" of the entire cabbage family. Kale resembles collards, except that its leaves are curly at the edges. When cooked, kale shrinks less than other greens and offers a stronger flavor and coarser texture. Your local grocer probably carries the deep-green variety, but kale also comes in yellow-green, red, or purple, with either flat or ruffled leaves.

Kale provides more nutritional value for fewer calories than almost any other food. A cup of kale serves up an abundance of manganese, a trace mineral that helps produce energy from protein and carbohydrates. Manganese is also a critical component of an essential antioxidant enzyme called superoxide dismutase, which provides important protection against free radicals. Kale supplies both vitamin B6 and riboflavin, a dynamic duo that protects lipids like cholesterol from being attacked—and damaged—by free radicals. The high fiber content of kale helps reduce cholesterol levels and keep blood sugar levels under control.

As a Fat Flush food, kale offers calcium for healthy bones, lutein to protect the eyes from cataracts, and indole-3-carbinol to guard against colon cancer, plus a healthy dose of iron, vitamin A, and vitamin C. Do yourself a favor by grabbing a supply of these superstar greens the next time you go shopping.

Recommended Usage

Daily as desired.

Just the Facts

- Kale is available year-round, but it is most tender and flavorful during the winter months.

- You may substitute kale for spinach in just about any recipe you like.
- One cup of kale provides over 200 percent more than the daily requirement of vitamin A and 75 percent of the daily need for vitamin C.
- While edible, colored varieties of kale, sometimes called salad Savoy, are most often grown for ornamental purposes. They do have a stronger flavor than regular kale.

Boost the Benefits

- Look for crisp, dark, bluish-green leaves that are not wilted, yellowing, or marked by tiny holes. The stems, which are edible, should be plump and moist.
- If you see kale with smaller-sized leaves, grab it up, because it is especially tender and offers a mild flavor. Coarse, oversized leaves are likely to be tough and bitter.
- To store kale, wrap it in a damp paper towel, place it in a perforated plastic bag, and keep it in the coldest part of the refrigerator. Washing it before you store it may cause it to become limp.
- Kale can be kept in the refrigerator for several days, although it is best when eaten within a day or two, since the longer it is stored, the stronger its flavor becomes. Even if the leaves still look nice and green, they will have an unpleasant taste after a day or two.
- To remove the sand and dirt from kale, wash it prior to cooking by swishing the separate leaves in a large basin of cool water. Lift the leaves from the water, let the sand and grit settle to the bottom, and repeat if necessary. Do not soak the leaves.

Be a Fat Flush Cook

- If the kale stems are thin and tender, just trim off the very tips and cook the stems along with the leaves. If the stems are tough, remove them by folding each leaf in half, vein-side out, and pulling up on the stem as you keep the leaf folded.
- You may use whole kale leaves if they are small, but it's best to strip the larger leaves from the center rib. To shred kale, place the leaves in a pile, roll them up together, and cut them into thin slices.
- Baby kale may be eaten raw and is delicious mixed with other greens in a salad.
- Mature kale is too tough to consume raw. You may steam, blanch, braise, sauté, or boil it. Depending on the method, cooking time varies from 5 to 30 minutes.
- Whenever possible, plan to use the cooking liquid from kale in a sauce or soup broth so that none of the nutrients are wasted.

- Try adding chopped kale to soups and stews.
- Braise chopped kale and apples. Before serving, sprinkle with apple cider vinegar and slivered almonds.

THINK TWICE!

- *Kale is among a small number of foods that contain oxalates, naturally occurring substances that can crystallize in the body and cause kidney stones. If you have been diagnosed with kidney or gallbladder problems, check with your physician before making kale a frequent menu item.*

IT'S BEEN SAID . . .

A huge serving of kale on my plate really fills me up and helps me maintain my thirty-pound weight loss. I love to sauté it in broth with some fresh garlic. Just before serving, I sprinkle it with some lemon juice and a dash of olive oil.

MAGGIE T., VERMONT

SPAGHETTI SQUASH

Fat Flush Factors
Blood-Sugar Stabilizer
Cholesterol Zapper

What vegetable looks like a small, yellow watermelon and can take the place of pasta at dinner? It's spaghetti squash, a variety of winter squash with mildly sweet flesh that pulls apart to form slender spaghetti-like strands. Averaging from four to eight pounds each, spaghetti squash can usually be found year-round and offers a bounty of nutritional benefits.

While research is ongoing, preliminary studies have shown that juice from squash has the ability to assist the body in fighting both cancer-like cell mutations and prostate problems. Beta-carotene, one of the most abundant nutrients in spaghetti squash, has powerful antioxidant and anti-inflammatory properties. It can prevent the oxidation of cholesterol in the body, regulate blood sugar levels, and thwart insulin resistance. The potassium found in spaghetti squash helps to lower blood pressure, and its fiber keeps cancer-causing chemicals from attacking colon cells.

As an added bonus, spaghetti squash is an excellent source of folate, which is needed by the body to break down a dangerous metabolic by-product called homocysteine. Since homocysteine can damage blood vessel walls, consuming plenty of folate can decrease your risk for heart attack and stroke. So while spaghetti squash has a hard shell that can be quite difficult to pierce, it is definitely worth the trouble.

Recommended Usage

At least one cup of spaghetti squash per week.

Just the Facts

- Vegetable spaghetti, vegetable marrow, spaghetti squash, noodle squash, and squaghetti are all names for this versatile vegetable.
- You'll end up with about five cups of "spaghetti" from the average four-pound squash.
- A spaghetti squash with a soft rind may be watery and lacking in flavor.
- Spaghetti squash with a dark orange color has more beta-carotene than squashes of the golden yellow variety.

Boost the Benefits

- At the store, look for a firm squash that is heavy for its size. The rind should have a dull sheen and a pale, even color. If the stem is still attached, it should be dry and rounded, not moist, shriveled, or blackened.
- Soft spots and green color are signs that the squash is not ripe. Moldy, water-soaked areas are indications of decay.
- Do not wash winter squash before storing it. Spaghetti squash can be stored at room temperature for about a month, but once you've cut into it, it will keep in the refrigerator for up to two days.
- Spaghetti squash freezes well. Pack cooked squash into freezer bags and toss them into the freezer. Before using, thaw the squash partially and then steam for about five minutes.

Be a Fat Flush Cook

- If you have trouble cutting through the shell of a spaghetti squash, try cooking it in a slow cooker. Select a squash that fits into your slow cooker. Pierce it several times with a large fork or skewer. Place it in the slow cooker and add two cups of water. Cover and cook on low for eight to nine hours. Cut in half and enjoy.
- Spaghetti squash can also be baked, boiled, or steamed. Once the squash is cooked, let it cool for 10 minutes before cutting it in half. Remove the seeds and pull a fork lengthwise through the flesh to separate it into long strands.
- Serve spaghetti squash with your favorite pasta sauce.
- Chill the squash strands and then toss them with your favorite Fat Flush dressing. Add some fresh tomato chunks, and you've got a refreshing—and beautiful—side dish.

IT'S BEEN SAID . . .

A great idea for leftover spaghetti squash is to mix in an egg, add whatever herbs and spices you like, ladle the mixture (by the ¼ cupful) into a hot skillet (coated with a quick spray of olive oil), and cook like pancakes. You can make this savory or sweet . . . my family loves theirs with cinnamon and Stevia.

LINDA S., FLORIDA

TOMATOES

Fat Flush Factors
Blood Sugar Stabilizer *Cholesterol Zapper* *Energizer*

A century ago, most Americans considered the tomato to be an odd, even poisonous, food. How times have changed. Today, sweet, juicy tomatoes are a staple in homes—and gardens—all across the United States. Tomatoes come in many different varieties. In addition to the "basic" tomato, your local grocery may carry petite cherry tomatoes, bright yellow tomatoes, Italian pear-shaped tomatoes, and the small green tomato, or tomatillo, common in Mexican fare.

Tomatoes are an excellent source of vitamins C and A, providing detoxifying antioxidants to neutralize dangerous free radicals that could otherwise damage cells and escalate problems with atherosclerosis, diabetic complications, asthma, and colon cancer. In addition, tomatoes supply fiber, which has been shown to lower cholesterol levels, control blood sugar levels, and help prevent colon cancer.

Tomatoes offer a trio of notable heart-healthy nutrients: potassium, vitamin B6, and folate. In addition, studies in the United States and Europe have concluded that lycopene, a phytonutrient found in tomatoes, lowers cholesterol levels and reduces the risk of heart disease. Tomatoes improve your body's energy production by supplying a bounty of biotin and help maintain bone health by serving as a source of vitamin K. And those blood sugar levels, already supported by the fiber in tomatoes, are stabilized even further by their chromium content.

Tomatoes are a marvelous vegetable loaded with an array of critical nutrients. By increasing your consumption of tomatoes, you'll take a big step forward toward flushing your fat and improving your health.

Recommended Usage
Daily as desired.

Just the Facts

• Although technically a fruit, tomatoes can't pass for dessert the way other fruits can. Their sweetness is subtle, toned down by a high acid content and slightly bitter flavor.

• The most concentrated source of vitamin C in a tomato is the jelly-like substance surrounding the seeds. But keep in mind that a hothouse-grown tomato has half the vitamin C content of a vine-ripened tomato.

• In France, the tomato is called a *pomme d'amour*, or "love apple," since it is believed to be an aphrodisiac.

• Combining tomatoes with bread or other starches creates an acidic reaction in the body, causing an upset stomach in some people. To avoid this, eat tomatoes alone or with other fresh vegetables.

Boost the Benefits

• Look for well-shaped, smooth tomatoes with no wrinkles, cracks, bruises, or soft spots. For the best flavor, select tomatoes with a deep, rich color. The deep color indicates that the fruit is loaded with the desirable antioxidant lycopene.

• Take a pass on puffy-looking tomatoes because they tend to be watery.

• Generally, the best-tasting tomatoes are the ones grown locally because they have been allowed to mature and ripen on the vine. Most local tomatoes contain twice as much vitamin C as tomatoes that were picked green or grown in a hothouse. Use your nose to check for a vine-ripened tomato. It should have a fresh, tomato smell, while a tomato that was picked green and then ripened artificially has a "gassy" or chemical smell.

• Store tomatoes at room temperature, away from direct sunlight. They will keep for up to a week, depending upon how ripe they are when they are purchased.

• To speed up the ripening process, place tomatoes in a paper bag along with an apple. The ethylene gas emitted by the apple will help mature the tomatoes.

• If the tomatoes ripen but you are not yet ready to eat them, place them in the refrigerator, where they will keep for a day or two. Remove them from the refrigerator about an hour before using them to allow for maximum flavor and juiciness.

• Whole tomatoes, chopped tomatoes, and tomato sauce freeze well, so don't be afraid to stock up when you find vine-ripened tomatoes.

• To get the greatest health benefits from the nutrients and the fiber, eat your tomatoes unpeeled.

Be a Fat Flush Cook

- If your recipe requires *seeded* tomatoes, cut the fruit in half horizontally and gently scoop the seeds out with a teaspoon.
- Add chopped tomatoes to your favorite vegetable soup recipe.
- Combine chopped onions, tomatoes, cumin, and cayenne for a super-easy salsa.
- Instead of a second piece of bread, top your sandwich with a couple of deep-red tomato slices.
- To prevent tomatoes from turning acidic, simmer them slowly rather than bringing them to a rolling boil.

THINK TWICE!

- *If you purchase canned tomatoes, check the label to make sure they were produced in the United States. Many foreign countries do not have high standards for lead content in cans. The high acid content of tomatoes can cause lead to leach into the can's contents.*
- *Avoid aluminum cookware when preparing tomatoes since their high acid content interacts with aluminum and may cause metal to leach into the food.*
- *If you hit a plateau when dieting, consider cutting down on your consumption of tomatoes. They rate a 25 on the glycemic index, while most of the other Fat Flush vegetables score less than 15. (The glycemic index ranks foods based on their immediate effect on your blood sugar. The lower the score, the less impact the food has on blood sugar levels.)*

Fat Flush Fun

A small boy was looking at the red ripe tomatoes growing in the farmer's garden.

"I'll give you my two pennies for that tomato," said the boy, pointing to a beautiful, large, ripe fruit hanging on the vine.

"No," said the farmer, "I get a dime for a tomato like that one."

The small boy pointed to a smaller green one.

"Will you take two pennies for that one?"

"Yes," replied the farmer, "I'll give you that one for two cents."

"OK," said the lad, sealing the deal by putting the coins in the farmer's hand, "I'll pick it up in about a week."

ITS' BEEN SAID . . .

I make my own Fat Flush spaghetti sauce by sautéing some fresh garlic in beef broth, adding chopped tomatoes and seasoning with my favorite herbs and spices. I let the mixture simmer until it has a rich, deep flavor. Then, I serve it over spaghetti squash for a fabulous Fat Flush meal!

JANET V., OKLAHOMA

WATERCRESS

Fat Flush Factors
Detoxifier
Diuretic

Watercress is the stuff legends are made of. According to Greek mythology, the god Zeus fortified himself against his enemies by eating watercress. In 460 BC, Hippocrates located his hospital near a stream so he would have access to fresh watercress, his treatment of choice for many ailments. And in nineteenth-century England, street vendors sold bunches of watercress as a handheld treat, to be eaten like an ice cream cone! So why do most people view watercress as mere garnish— a touch of green to decorate the plate?

Perhaps it's the pungent flavor, which is reminiscent of mustard, but with a refreshing, rather than fiery "bite" that makes watercress something of an acquired taste. If you have yet to make the acquaintance of this Fat Flush vegetable, consider adding it to your grocery list. Watercress is still grown using traditional gravel beds fed by fresh flowing spring water, and it contains a bounty of blood-purifying phytonutrients.

One such beneficial nutrient is the anticancer compound phenylethyl isothiocyanate, or PEITC. Whenever it is crushed, chopped, or chewed, watercress releases a peppery flavor, evidence of the PEITC content. The more pungent the taste, the more PEITC is being released, and the greater the health benefit.

In addition, watercress contains generous amounts of vitamins A and C, along with hefty doses of calcium, folic acid, potassium, and iron. Regular consumption of watercress boosts kidney efficiency and does away with hunger pangs. Best of all, watercress is a superb natural diuretic, serving as a powerful Fat Flush tool for reducing water retention and bloating.

Recommended Usage

At least one bunch of watercress per week.

Just the Facts

• Watercress is a fantastic source of vitamin C and, ounce for ounce, contains more iron than spinach and more calcium than milk.
• Watercress can grow anywhere there is running water.
• The Chinese eat ten times more watercress than Americans do, often tossing two or three bunches into one stir-fried dish.

Boost the Benefits

• Look for glossy, dark-green watercress leaves and crisp stems.
• Typically, young watercress contains less mustard oil than older watercress but is easier to digest, allowing the body to get the most benefit from the phytonutrients.
• Watercress should be kept moist with damp paper towels, wrapped in plastic, and stored in the refrigerator. It will keep this way for about a week.
• If necessary, revitalize watercress by submerging it in ice water, discarding any wilted, bruised, or yellow leaves.

Be a Fat Flush Cook

• Use watercress like you would any lettuce, giving the stems a slight trim.
• Toss fresh watercress leaves into a mixture of fat-flushing berries. Top with a squeeze of lemon juice for a delicious dessert idea.
• Watercress and ginger combine well in any stir-fry dish.
• Add chopped watercress to your next omelet.
• Cooking mellows the mustardy bite of watercress, making it a fantastic addition to any soup. You can also steam it as a side dish for fish or poultry.

IT'S BEEN SAID . . .

The eating of watercress doth restore the wanted bloom to the cheeks of old-young ladies.

LORD FRANCIS BACON, ENGLISH PHILOSOPHER

ZUCCHINI

Fat Flush Factors

Cholesterol Zapper
Detoxifier

Probably the best known of the summer squashes, the zucchini is a cousin to both the melon and the cucumber. Native to America, it was brought back to Europe by Christopher Columbus. Today, zucchini is grown and enjoyed around the world, especially between May and July, when it is most abundant.

Zucchini's creamy white flesh has a delicate flavor, but the entire vegetable is edible and nutritious, including its flesh, skin, and seeds. Zucchini is a good source of vitamins A, B6, and C and potassium, magnesium, folate, riboflavin, and fiber; many of these nutrients help prevent atherosclerosis and diabetic heart disease. The magnesium in zucchini reduces the risk of heart attack and stroke, while the potassium brings down high blood pressure. The vitamin C and beta-carotene found in zucchini help prevent the oxidation of cholesterol, keeping atherosclerosis at bay. And zucchini's vitamin B6 and folate are used to break down homocysteine, a substance that contributes to heart disease.

The nutrients in zucchini offer valuable protection against other diseases as well. The high fiber content of zucchini absorbs cancer-causing toxins, keeping them away from cells in the colon. The beta-carotene found in zucchini has anti-inflammatory properties that fight conditions such as asthma, arthritis, and irritable bowel syndrome. During your next trip to the supermarket, load up on these lean, green, disease-fighting veggies.

Recommended Usage

Daily as desired.

Just the Facts

- Generally, one medium-sized zucchini serves one person.
- Zucchini is the most popular of the summer squashes and the only vegetable that begins with the letter *z*.

- The flavor of zucchini is sweetest when it is less than 6 inches long. Zucchinis can grow as large as baseball bats, but when they reach this size, they have little flavor and large, tough seeds.

Boost the Benefits

- When you're shopping, look for zucchinis that are firm, glossy, and heavy for their size. The skin should be smooth, without bruises, and deep green in color.
- Beware a zucchini with a hard rind, since it is probably past its prime and will have hard seeds and stringy flesh.
- Handle zucchini with care, since it is very fragile and small punctures will lead to decay.
- Store zucchini in a breathable plastic bag in the refrigerator for up to one week. Be sure the zucchini is dry when you put it in the bag, because moisture generates mold and spoilage.
- To retain maximum vitamins and fiber, do not peel zucchini.

Be a Fat Flush Cook

- Onion and garlic go well with zucchini, but you can add flavor to zucchini by experimenting with any of the Fat Flush herbs and spices.
- Zucchini's mild flavor blends well with plain yogurt, lemon, olive oil, peppers, mushrooms, or onions.
- Steaming is a great way to prepare zucchini; the finished product is sweet and crisp. You can also grill it, toss it in a stir-fry, or munch on it raw.
- Experiment with zucchini by grating it or cutting it into sticks or rings or make zucchini into "zoodles" with a spiralizer if you are grain-free.
- If you overcook zucchini, you'll end up with mush. If that should happen to you, your best bet is to toss the mushy zucchini in some soup!

THINK TWICE!

- *People who have been diagnosed with kidney or gallbladder problems may want to avoid eating zucchini on a regular basis since it contains oxalates, a substance that can crystallize in the body and cause kidney stones.*
- *If you cut into a zucchini and immediately notice an acrid odor, do not eat it! There have been rare cases in which a compound called cucurbitacin E has been found in zucchini. It creates extreme bitterness in a zucchini. In addition to the unpleasant smell and bitter flavor, this compound can cause cramps and diarrhea.*

IT'S BEEN SAID . . .

Who needs potato chips or pretzels? I love to snack on zucchini chips, made by baking thin slices of zucchini in a 350 degree oven for about 15 minutes.

THOMAS D., MARYLAND

4 Fat Flush Fruits

Some things you have to do every day. Eating seven apples on Saturday night instead of one a day just isn't going to get the job done.

—JIM ROHN

The Fat Flush approach to fruits is sure to be controversial. Sure, fruits are Mother Nature's candy and provide a healthy way to satisfy your sweet tooth while filling up on Fat Flush vitamins, minerals, enzymes, and fiber. But the sugar found in fruits—fructose—when taken in excess has been linked to obesity, type 2 diabetes, fatty liver, high triglycerides and uric acid, GI problems, and accelerated aging. So the fruits that have received the Fat Flush seal of approval are the lowest in fructose and need to be enjoyed in designated quantities (1 cup berries, 1 small apple, 10 cherries, ½ banana, and so on) so you don't overdo too much of a good thing.

Now that we have that nutritional bombshell out of the way, let's talk about all the wonderful benefits fruits bestow. Because they contain a high percentage of water, fruits help hydrate the body, while, at the same time, their impressive levels of potassium and magnesium work to wring excess water weight from body tissues. Cellulose, the fibrous matter in fruits, provides smooth passage for food in the digestive tract and eases bowel action. This laxative effect is enhanced by the sugar and organic acids in fruit.

Many fruits contain phytochemicals, compounds that help prevent chronic diseases such as cardiovascular disease, cancer, and diabetes. Fruits are also famous for their antioxidants, which slow down oxidation and prevent cell and tissue damage. Countless studies have shown that eating a variety of fruits helps control blood pressure; prevent heart attacks, strokes, and cancer; and even maintain eye health.

Fruits have what it takes to maintain the body's acid-alkaline balance. In fact, the vitamins, minerals, and enzymes in fruits are extremely beneficial in normalizing all the body's processes. What researchers have discovered is that while fruits contain a number of nutritious elements, it is the *combined* power of all the nutrients working together that gives fruits their disease-fighting abilities. Fat Flush fruits are a must for a healthy, balanced diet. It's easy to fit them into most any meal, especially your morning smoothies—or save them for snack time since they are best digested on an empty stomach.

APPLES

Fat Flush Factors

Blood Sugar Stabilizer
Cholesterol Zapper
Detoxifier

Whether its peel is red, yellow, or green, few things are as refreshing as the crisp, white flesh of an apple. From Adam and Eve to Johnny Appleseed, apples have played an important part in history and mythology. Originally from eastern Europe and Asia, the apple is one of the oldest cultivated fruits. Certain varieties of apples have been grown for at least 2,000 years, and over the centuries, people have developed more than 7,000 varieties of apple.

From the crisp, aromatic Braeburn to the green tang of a Granny Smith, apples contain a number of components, namely fiber and flavonoids, that lower cholesterol, improve bowel function, and reduce the risk of heart disease, stroke, cancer, diabetes, and asthma! The research on apples is extensive and varied. The National Cancer Institute reported that flavonoids, a type of antioxidant found in apples, may reduce the risk of lung cancer by up to 50 percent. A group of researchers at the University of California at Davis found that two apples a day may decrease oxidation of LDL cholesterol by up to 34 percent. And quercetin, a potent flavonoid found in apple peel, has been shown to reduce the risk of heart attack by 32 percent.

Offering both soluble and insoluble fiber, apples are known for aiding digestion and promoting weight loss. Even though they are rich in natural sugar, apples do not cause a rapid rise in blood sugar levels. The nutritional makeup of the apple prevents the body from pumping out too much insulin. In addition, apples contain a natural fibrous chemical called pectin, which limits the amount of fat absorbed by your cells. Pectin also grabs toxins, such as the heavy metals lead and mercury, and escorts them out of the body. Studies have shown that because of their pectin, green apples are the best choice for cleansing the liver.

Pectin prevails over the appetite, too. Researchers at Texas's Brooke Army Medical Center studied the impact of pectin on hunger by feeding orange juice to a group of 74 people. Half the people got plain orange juice, and half got juice with added pectin. People who received the pectin-laced juice reported having little sense of hunger for four hours, while the people who drank regular orange juice complained of hunger much sooner. The researchers concluded that pectin may slow digestion, keeping food in the stomach longer. So whether you grab an apple as a snack or serve it as a delicious dessert, you'll be cleansing your body and trimming your waistline at the same time.

Recommended Usage

An apple a day.

Just the Facts

- While Washington is famous for its apple orchards, apples are grown in almost every state in the United States.
- The average American eats about 120 apples every year—a far cry from an apple a day!
- Did you ever wonder why it's customary to give an apple to a teacher? This practice began when public school teachers were paid in food or goods, rather than money.
- Researchers at Yale University discovered that some people lowered their blood pressure just by smelling the pleasant scent of spiced apples.

Boost the Benefits

- When you're buying apples, select fruit that is firm, richly colored, and free of soft spots.
- In the Northern Hemisphere, apple season begins at the end of summer and lasts until early winter. When you buy apples at other times of the year, they have been imported from the Southern Hemisphere.
- Skip the apple juice and go for the whole apple instead. It provides more nutrition and fiber than the juice.
- To prevent further ripening, store apples in a plastic bag in the refrigerator. They should stay fresh for up to six weeks, but it's a good idea to check them regularly and remove any apples that begin to decay before they affect the others.
- Protect apple slices from oxidation and discoloration by dipping them into a solution of one part lemon juice and three parts water.

Be a Fat Flush Cook

- An apple is the perfect portable snack. Experiment with different varieties throughout the year.
- The tarter the apple, the better it maintains its texture during cooking.
- Add diced apples to tossed green salads if your digestion can tolerate both fruits and veggies at the same time.
- Simmer a chopped apple in broth with red cabbage or combine a Granny Smith in your butternut squash soup.

THINK TWICE!

- *Commercially raised apples may have been exposed to as many as 10 pesticides. You can avoid consuming these pesticides by removing the skin, but you will be sacrificing both fiber and flavonoids, so go organic.*

IT'S BEEN SAID . . .

I was looking for a Fat Flush alternative to sweet desserts, so I sliced an apple and shook the slices in a plastic bag with a tablespoon of ground flax seed and half a teaspoon of cinnamon. Having this treat in the evening has helped me stick to the Fat Flush Plan—and lose 25 pounds!

SANDY M., CALIFORNIA

Comfort me with apples for I am sick.

KING SOLOMON, THE BIBLE

BANANAS

Fat Flush Factors
Blood Sugar Stabilizer
Detoxifier
Energizer

Bananas are probably the most popular fruit on the planet. Very few natural foods come off the tree already packaged for busy people on the go! The banana is one of the oldest cultivated plants, used for millennia as a remedy for everything from upset stomach to constipation, dysentery, PMS, hemorrhoids, warts, and many other maladies.

Technically, bananas are a berry. They do contain seeds, but the seeds are so small they go unnoticed. Bananas are rich in potassium and magnesium—two nutrients known to lower your risk for heart attack and stroke, as well as preventing muscle cramps. Potassium helps lower blood pressure. One banana contains 467 milligrams of potassium, which is about 9 percent of the recommended daily allowance.

In terms of sugar, the beloved banana is a bit toward the high end. A cup of banana slices (one largish banana) contains about 18 grams of sugar, compared with 13 grams for apples and 8 grams for strawberries. This is why bananas are not allowed on phase 1 of my New Fat Flush Plan. However, this doesn't mean bananas in moderation are not a good part of a lifestyle plan, once your metabolism is optimized.

Bananas are high in several antioxidants, which reduce free-radical damage and lower your risk for most chronic diseases, including cancer. They contain significant flavonoids such as lutein, zeaxanthin, and alpha- and beta-carotenes, as well as being a great source of vitamin C, B6, manganese, copper, iron, L-tryptophan, choline, and fiber. L-tryptophan is an amino acid that gets converted to 5-HTP in your brain, which in turn is converted to serotonin and melatonin. So a banana at bedtime may help you sleep!

The flavonoids are good for your eyes. The choline (12 milligrams per banana) has abundant benefits throughout your body, including reducing abdominal fat storage.

The starch in bananas deserves special mention. Bananas—especially unripe bananas—contain a special type of "resistant starch" that has fabulous benefits for your health. Fructooligosaccharides (or FOS) are fibers that resist digestion in your small intestine and slowly ferment in your large intestine. These special starches act as prebiotics for feeding the friendly bacteria. They also bulk up your stools, won't make you gassy, and aren't likely to trigger blood sugar spikes like so many other starches. Bananas also contain pectin, which is beneficial for digestion and detoxification.

Research shows that FOS (resistant starch) improves insulin regulation and blood glucose levels and slows stomach emptying, which improves satiety. FOS is also known to increase your body's absorption of calcium, which is good news for your bones.

If you're going to eat bananas, go for the green! Unripe bananas have much higher FOS levels than ripe ones because the starch is converted into sugar during ripening. Before ripening, a banana is almost entirely starch, making up 70 to 80 percent by weight—and a large part of this is resistant starch. The FOS in green bananas is why they've been used for centuries to treat diarrhea. By the way, the idea that bananas cause constipation is a myth. A 2011 study concluded that not only do bananas *not* cause constipation, but they increase beneficial Bifidobacteria in your gut. Participants consuming bananas reported reduced digestive complaints including bloating and stomach pain.

A few studies have revealed even more interesting health benefits. A Swedish study found that women who ate bananas two to three times per week were 33 percent less likely to develop kidney disease. Another study found that children who ate one banana daily showed 34 percent less risk for asthma. Yet another study showed that endurance cyclists who ate half a banana every 15 minutes during a 3-hour race maintained energy levels equal to those of cyclists who drank sports drinks.

So although bananas are notoriously high in sugar, they also contain a boatload of valuable nutrients. The sugar issue is somewhat mitigated by the presence of FOS, which you can increase by eating bananas that are less ripe.

Recommended Usage

- Bananas are allowed in phase 2 of my New Fat Flush Plan.
- Slice up bananas and keep them in the freezer for a quick addition to your smoothies.

Just the Facts

- Along with plantains, the banana plant belongs to the Musaceae family and grows to an impressive 10 to 26 feet. Today, bananas grow in most tropical and subtropical zones, with the main commercial producers being Mexico, Costa Rica, Ecuador, and Brazil.

- Bananas are thought to have originated in Malaysia around 4,000 years ago before being transported by early explorers to India and the Philippines.
- Bananas contain antihistamines; rubbing an insect bite or hives with the inside of a banana peel may relieve itching. It is said that a wart can be cured by taping a piece of banana peel against it.
- Do bananas make you feel good? If so, it might be because of the neurotransmitters they contain—norepinephrine, dopamine, and serotonin.
- The peel and pulp of fully ripe bananas have antifungal and antibiotic properties; the antibiotic is effective against Mycobacteria.

Boost the Benefits

- Look for organic bananas. Many conventional banana plantations utilize chemical fertilizers and aerial spraying of pesticides.
- Green bananas take longer to ripen than those with more yellow or a few brown spots. If you want your green bananas to ripen, leave them at room temperature, because putting them in the fridge will irreversibly disrupt the ripening process.
- Ripe bananas that you don't plan to consume for a few days can be stored in the refrigerator. The peel will darken but the flesh will not be affected.
- You can freeze bananas whole, sliced, or as a puree. Frozen bananas will keep for a couple of months.

THINK TWICE!

- *Certain medications used for heart disease and hypertension, such as beta-blockers, have the potential to increase potassium levels, so high-potassium foods should be consumed in moderation. Potassium imbalances (hyperkalemia and hypokalemia) are serious and can lead to deadly heart arrhythmias.*
- *Consuming too many potassium-rich foods can be harmful for those with compromised kidney function.*

Fat Flush Fun

- Green banana flour is now being used to make gluten-free pasta.
- The things for which banana peels have been put to use are numerous—everything from relieving hemorrhoids to polishing silverware, shining leather shoes, removing splinters, whitening teeth, and perk-

ing up the leaves of lackluster house plants. Did you know that banana peels can be used to make vinegar?

- A fungicide in the peel and pulp of green bananas is active against a fungus that afflicts tomato plants.
- According to *Medical News Today,* minced banana peels performed better than anything else tested for water purification.
- There is a superstition that bananas are "unlucky" aboard fishing boats and will bring all sorts of misfortune such as preventing the fish from biting, causing the boat to sink, harboring poisonous spiders, or giving off methane gas and thereby killing the crew. To this day, many seafaring captains prohibit bringing bananas aboard their ships. These superstitions appear to have originated on the banana boats of the Caribbean trade of the 1700s.

BERRIES

Fat Flush Factors
Cholesterol Zapper
Detoxifier
Energizer

While there are many types of berries—from smooth-skinned varieties to those with fleshy segments—I am focusing on three Fat Flush favorites: raspberries, strawberries, and blueberries. Raspberries can be traced back to prehistoric times, strawberries have grown wild around the world for thousands of years, and blueberries are native to North America.

Filled with the antioxidant ellagic acid, raspberries help prevent damage to cell membranes by neutralizing free radicals. Raspberries also contain flavonoids, the substances that give them their rich red color. These phytonutrients prevent overgrowth of bacteria and fungi, including *Candida albicans*—a factor in yeast infections and those pesky carb cravings. Brimming with manganese, vitamin C, a number of B vitamins, and dietary fiber, raspberries benefit the liver by cleansing the blood.

Strawberries reign supreme as the most popular berry in America. They contain the most vitamin C of any berry and plenty of cancer-protective ellagic acid. Phytonutrients called anthocyanins give strawberries their inviting red color while packing a potent fat-flushing punch by breaking down excess toxins in the liver.

As researchers at Tufts University discovered, blueberries provide more antioxidants—including the powerful cholesterol fighter resveratrol—than most other common fruits or vegetables. They contain significant amounts of both antibacterial and antiviral compounds, and they may also protect against heart disease and cancer. High in fiber, blueberries also contain tannins, which serve to cleanse the digestive system. And they promote a healthy urinary tract by preventing bacterial growth.

All berries are bursting with vitamin C, which stimulates production of carnitine, an amino acid that boosts metabolism. In addition, berries contain natural fructose, which is satisfying to a sweet tooth. Researchers have also found that the insoluble fiber in berries prevents their total calories from being absorbed, making them a tasty Fat Flush treat!

Recommended Usage

Add a handful of berries to your daily diet.

Just the Facts

- Across the United States, fresh blueberries are available for nearly eight months of the year.
- If all the blueberries grown annually in North America were spread out in a single layer, they would cover a four-lane highway stretching from New York to Chicago.
- Until the 1800s, strawberries remained a luxury food, found only in the kitchens of the wealthy.
- Strawberries are not considered a "true" berry, because they grow from the base of the plant rather than from a flower ovary.
- Currently, the strawberry is the most popular berry in the world, with blueberries coming in a close second.
- If a raspberry's green "cap" is intact, the berry is immature and will never become sweet.

Boost the Benefits

- When you're buying berries, look for plump, firm fruits with a deep, shiny color. Shake the container to see if the berries move freely. If not, the berries may be soft, damaged, or moldy.
- Keep in mind that moisture causes berries to decay. Stay away from berry containers that are stained or wet.
- When purchasing frozen berries, shake the bag gently to check for freely moving berries. If the fruit seems clumped together, the bag may have been thawed and refrozen. Properly handled, frozen berries should keep for about a year.
- Always check berries before storing and remove any damaged berries to prevent the spread of mold.
- Berries may be stored in a covered container in the refrigerator for about three to five days. However, for optimal health benefits and flavor, plan to serve berries within a day or two after purchasing them.
- Fresh berries—especially raspberries—are very fragile and should be washed briefly and carefully and then gently patted dry. To preserve the texture and flavor of strawberries, wash them *before* you remove their caps.
- You'll notice the fullest flavor if you eat fresh berries at room temperature.

Be a Fat Flush Cook

- Add color and flavor to a mixed green salad by tossing in some sliced strawberries.
- A few ripe raspberries make a beautiful (and delicious) garnish for a salad or dessert.
- Layer sliced strawberries, whole blueberries, and plain yogurt in a wine glass to make a parfait dessert.
- Fresh or frozen berries make a perfect addition to a Fat Flush whey protein smoothie.
- A few luscious frozen strawberries make a refreshing and revitalizing summer snack.

PEACHES

Fat Flush Factors
Detoxifier
Diuretic

Originally from China, peaches have captivated Americans since well before Thomas Jefferson planted 160 peach trees in his orchard. Today, nearly 300 varieties of this succulent fruit thrive in warm climates around the world.

There are two categories of peaches: clingstone and freestone. They are differentiated by how easily the fruit pulls away from the pit. With freestones, the pit comes away easily, but with cling peaches, separating the pit is more of a challenge.

Peaches are high in the antioxidant vitamins A and C, which promote beautiful, ageless skin, healthy vision, and a strong immune system. This fuzzy fruit is also a good source of potassium, fiber, and beta cryptothanxin, a phytonutrient recognized for preventing heart disease. And while peaches are already known to prevent certain types of cancer, new varieties of the fruit are being developed that will yield even higher levels of cancer-fighting antioxidants and phytochemicals.

Peaches have both a diuretic and a laxative effect and help stimulate digestive juices. This nutritious Fat Flush fruit also contains boron, known to pump up estrogen levels in postmenopausal women, stimulate the brain, and help prevent osteoporosis. So feel free to indulge in a juicy ripe peach whenever you like. It only tastes sinful.

Recommended Usage

Three or four peaches per week.

Just the Facts

- Usually, freestone peaches are sold fresh, while clingstones are canned, frozen, and preserved.
- In ancient China, people believed that the peach conferred immortality on those who ate it. Today, the peach remains a symbol of hope and longevity.

- To pit a peach easily, slice it horizontally all the way around and then twist the halves apart.
- Because of consumer demand, peaches aren't as fuzzy as they used to be. After being picked, most peaches are mechanically brushed to get rid of some of the fuzz.

Boost the Benefits

- When you're shopping for peaches, go for unblemished fruit that is free of bruises and that has a warm, fragrant aroma.
- Contrary to popular belief, the red blush on peaches is not a measure of ripeness. Instead, look for peaches with a creamy or golden under-color and pass on peaches with a greenish color. They were picked before they matured and will *never* ripen.
- To test for ripeness, squeeze a peach gently. A peach is prime when it gives to slight pressure and smells sweet.
- If you need to ripen peaches, store them in a loosely closed brown bag at room temperature. Never store fresh peaches in plastic bags. This changes their flavor and texture.
- You can store ripe peaches in the crisper bin of your refrigerator for a few days, but they may lose some of their flavor. Whenever possible, bring them to room temperature before serving.
- Keep in mind that most of a peach's vitamins are in the peel, so eat the whole peach, fuzz and all, whenever possible.

Be a Fat Flush Cook

- Try poaching peaches and serving them as a simple dessert.
- Add peach chunks to a skewer of meat and vegetables for grilling.
- Pop some peach slices into a blender with some cranberry juice, whey protein, and spices for a satisfying breakfast smoothie.
- Peaches may be baked, grilled, or broiled and served along with your favorite meat or fish dinner.
- For a quick and easy dessert, slice a fresh peach and then top it with a dollop of plain yogurt and a sprinkling of cinnamon and ground flax seed.

THINK TWICE!

- *Peach pits contain a toxic substance known as hydrocyanic acid, or cyanide, and can be fatal if ingested in large quantities. So be sure to dispose of the pits properly to keep them away from children and pets.*

PINEAPPLE

Fat Flush Factors
Detoxifier
Energizer

What if there were a food that gave you radiant skin and tons of energy while at the same time soothing joint pain and busting up cellulite? That's exactly what you get from pineapple! This big, spiny-looking fruit has been a coveted part of traditional Hawaiian medicine for generations, used to treat indigestion, joint pain, allergies, and much more.

Second only to bananas as America's favorite tropical fruit, pineapple boasts a lovely array of vitamins, minerals, and phytonutrients, plus one uniquely powerful player: bromelain. Bromelain is a protein-digesting enzyme with potent anti-inflammatory effects and tremendous healing power. The enzyme offers benefits for a large number of diseases, and pineapple is our richest natural source—especially the stem and core.

Bromelain calms the pain and swelling of arthritis, reduces asthma and sinus symptoms, and quiets inflammatory bowel disease. It soothes the inflamed tissues of sprained ankles and tendonitis and helps heal ACL tears. In a 2014 study, bromelain was found to relieve pain among osteoarthritis sufferers by 50 to 60 percent. Bromelain also reduces phlegm and mucus buildup, which helps explain its benefits for respiratory conditions. In fact, bromelain helps modulate your entire immune system, making the enzyme beneficial for allergies and autoimmune issues as well. It also acts as an anticoagulant.

Bromelain has an additional feature that will excite anyone fighting the fat battle: it boosts fat metabolism and helps melt away cellulite. Bromelain dissolves waste and toxins trapped inside fat cells, allowing your lymph system to flush them away. This miracle enzyme also neutralizes bradykinins—polypeptides that promote fat storage on your hips and thighs.

Adding to all of this, bromelain has anticancer benefits. A 2014 study showed that it prompts the self-destruction of malignant peritoneal mesothelioma cells, a rare form of cancer caused by asbestos exposure. Bromelain has shown similar defenses against cancers of the mouth, throat, breast, colon, and lung.

Pineapples have benefits beyond bromelain. They're brimming with vitamin C, which is a great addition in the anticellulite department, as it helps rebuild collagen. Collagen is what gives your skin structure, and its breakdown is responsible, at least in part, for cellulite's lumpy appearance. Collagen is also essential for healthy organ tissues, bones, and blood vessels. One cup of fresh pineapple has 131 percent of the U.S. RDA for immune-boosting vitamin C.

You'll also find significant amounts of copper (which aids the formation of healthy red blood cells), vitamins B1 and B6, folate, pantothenic acid, antioxidants, and beta-carotene. Manganese is pineapple's most prominent mineral, with a single serving delivering over 70 percent of your RDA. Manganese helps build superoxide dismutase, a powerful free-radical scavenger. When it comes to this magical fruit, what's not to love?

Recommended Usage

* Due to pineapple's loftier sugar content, eat it in moderation. You'll take less of a sugar hit eating the whole fruit as opposed to drinking the juice, as the fiber will slow down absorption. If you do juice pineapple, cut its juice with low-sugar vegetable juices, like cucumber and celery.
* Eat pineapple on an empty stomach to take full advantage of its anti-inflammatory properties. However, if you're needing digestive help, then take it with food.

Just the Facts

* Pineapple did not originate in Hawaii but rather in Paraguay. Pineapple was spread from its native habitat by local Indians who carried it up through the South and Central Americas and to the West Indies. Then in the late 1400s, European explorers reportedly discovered pineapples on the Caribbean island known as Guadalupe.
* It is also reported that Columbus brought pineapples to Spain from the Americas in 1493, at the same time that European sailors spread it to the rest of the world by carrying it on ships in order to protect themselves from scurvy.
* The pineapple got its name in the seventeenth century due to its similarity in appearance to pine cones.
* The bulk of the world's pineapples now come from Southeast Asia, with Thailand being the largest producer.

Boost the Benefits

* Select a pineapple that's firm, heavy for its size, and devoid of bruising or soft spots. Choose one with a fragrant, sweet smell at the stem end and avoid any that have a musty, sour, or fermented smell.

- The healthiest part of the pineapple is its core, which contains most of the bromelain. The flesh is also nutritious, but it doesn't have the high bromelain content. The riper the fruit, the softer the core will be. Because of its toughness, the pineapple's core is easiest to consume juiced or blended into your smoothie.
- Although it does soften a little, pineapple stops ripening once it is picked; therefore, whole or cut pineapple should be stored in your fridge. Pineapple will keep for a couple of days on the counter or up to nine days in the fridge if properly wrapped. Freezing pineapple is OK from a nutritional standpoint, but freezing does affect its flavor.

Fat Flush in Action

- Prepare fresh pineapple by first placing your fruit on a large cutting board. Chop off the top and bottom ends using a large, sharp knife. Then trim off the rind and slice your fruit into rings.
- The area nearest the base of the fruit has more sugar, a sweeter taste, and a more tender texture.
- Pineapple is a phase 2 fruit. It pairs nicely with banana, mango, avocado, and coconut—and even a jalapeño for a zippy tropical fruit salsa.
- Pineapple chopped with fennel and cashews makes a lovely side dish for chicken.
- Replace sugar or liquid sweeteners with pineapple juice when making your own granola or baked goods.

THINK TWICE!

- *Bromelain is a meat-tenderization enzyme, and as such it can irritate your lips, gums, and tongue if you consume too much.*
- *Be cautious with pineapple if you are taking blood thinners due to its anticoagulant properties.*

Fat Flush Fun

- The pineapple's botanical name is *Ananas comosus*, belonging to the Bromeliaceae family.
- A pineapple is actually a composite of 100 to 200 coalesced "fruitlets" fused together at the crown of a fruit-bearing tree. Each fruitlet can be identified by an "eye"—the eyes are those prickly projections on the surface of a pineapple.
- Pineapple leaves are used in some parts of the world for wallpaper and ceiling insulation.

- You might grow your own pineapple plant at home! Just twist off the crown of a store-bought pineapple, dry it for a few days, and then plant it. Now you'll have to be patient . . . it takes two years for the plant to produce a single pineapple. But in the wild, pineapple plants can produce fruit for as long as 50 years.

POMEGRANATE

Fat Flush Factors
Blood Sugar Stabilizer *Cholesterol Zapper* *Detoxifier*

Pomegranate is a nutrient-packed fruit that shares many similar health benefits with the noble cranberry. Pomegranates have been the focus of a myriad of studies for their abundant health-giving properties, including support for your liver, detoxification, and weight management. A 2016 study found that in just 30 days, pomegranate extract was able to decrease blood glucose and insulin levels, reduce oxidative damage and inflammation, and substantially improve metabolic profiles in overweight and obese individuals.

The slightly six-sided pomegranate is the fruit of the shrub *Punica granatum*. Botanically, the pomegranate is a berry, but inside it's like nothing else . . . chambers upon chambers of hundreds of "arils," the term used for those juicy ruby-red pods you recognize as pomegranate seeds. The seeds are actually inside those tasty pods. A single pomegranate can hold more than 600 arils! They can be eaten raw or pressed into pomegranate juice. Pomegranates (the peel as well as the arils) contain substantial amounts of vitamin C, vitamin K, fiber, potassium, folate, vitamin B6, and phosphorous.

Pomegranates contain three types of antioxidant polyphenols: tannins, anthocyanins, and ellagic acid, with the most notable being punicalagins and punicalins. Punicic acid, also known as pomegranate seed oil, is the main fatty acid in the arils and is actually a type of conjugated linoleic acid. This special polyphenol potion offers three times the antioxidant punch of red wine or green tea.

Due to its over-the-top antioxidant action, the pomegranate offers outstanding protection for your heart, even in relatively small quantities—like two to four ounces per day. Science has identified substantial cardiovascular benefits including blood pressure stabilization, less platelet aggregation, and reduced arterial plaque and LDL oxidation. The same anti-inflammatory agents that benefit your heart also benefit the rest of your body, providing relief from arthritis, joint pain, and gastrointestinal maladies including ulcers.

Evidence shows pomegranates can improve memory in the elderly, as well as in anyone experiencing postsurgical memory impairment, and may offer some protection from Alzheimer's disease—again, stemming from those powerful polyphenols. Punicic acid has been shown to inhibit the spread of cancer, including breast, prostate, and other types. The pomegranate has antibacterial and antiviral effects, helps prevent bone loss, and even shows promise as a natural treatment for erectile dysfunction—which likely explains why the pomegranate has been long touted as an aphrodisiac.

Although pomegranate juice has a powerful array of nutrients, I challenge your inner adventurer to try out the fresh arils, allowing you to take full advantage of the fiber and live phytonutrients as well.

Recommended Usage

- There are a number of methods to go about liberating the seeds (arils) from the inside of a pomegranate. The Pomegranate Council recommends this simple three-step process:
  - Cut off the crown; then cut the pomegranate into sections.
  - Place each section in a bowl of water; then roll out the arils with your fingers (discard everything else).
  - Strain out the water and enjoy the arils. Inside each aril is a crunchy fiber-rich seed that is entirely edible.

Just the Facts

- Pomegranates have been used in traditional medicine to treat digestive problems, including combating intestinal parasites.
- Pomegranate powders and extracts are usually made from pomegranate peel.
- In North America, pomegranate season is generally September through December. The fruit grows in hotter, drier parts of the United States such as the Southwest.
- The pomegranate was introduced to California by Spanish settlers in 1769. Pomegranate trees can live as long as 300 years—so some of the original plants may still be around today!
- Pomegranates are native to the Middle East, and ancient Egyptians were often buried with them. Pomegranate is one of the seven spices (*shivat haminim*), seven fruits, and grains listed in the Hebrew Bible as native to Israel. The world's largest pomegranates grow in Kandahar, Afghanistan.
- In Hinduism, pomegranates symbolize fertility and prosperity. Pomegranates are incorporated into Persian wedding ceremonies to ensure a joyous future. In Greek mythology, however, pomegranates are a symbol of death . . . poor goddess Persephone was condemned to

spend every winter in the underworld after the god Hades tricked her into eating pomegranate seeds.
• The Spanish city Granada is named after the Spanish word for pomegranate, *granada*.

Boost the Benefits

• Whole pomegranates can be stored at room temperature for about a week. However, whole pomegranates will last up to two months if wrapped and stored in the refrigerator.
• Fresh pomegranate seeds can be refrigerated for up to three days, but frozen they'll keep for six months. Freeze arils on a tray, in a single layer, and then store in an airtight container. When thawed, they will be a bit shriveled but they do maintain their flavor.

Be a Fat Flush Cook

• Use pomegranate seeds for snacking, or sprinkle them over your yogurt, oatmeal, or chia seed pudding. Eat the whole seeds, little pits and all—that's where the fiber is!
• Add pomegranate seeds to salads, brussels sprouts, winter squash, or even quinoa. Add them to anything for a splash of color and a deluge of nutrition.
• Make "pomegranate molasses" by simmering down pomegranate juice into a thick syrup and then storing it in your fridge in an airtight glass jar. Now you have a "secret ingredient" for sauces, dressings, and marinades—or just a drizzle of happiness.
• How about some pomegranate sorbet?

THINK TWICE!

• *Pomegranate has been reported to sometimes produce significant interactions with certain medications, such as the blood thinner warfarin (Coumadin, Jantoven), and angiotensin-converting enzyme inhibitors such as captopril (Capoten), enalapril (Vasotec), and lisinopril (Prinivil, Zestril). Consult your physician before consuming pomegranate products if you take any of these medications.*
• *Pomegranate juice can really stain surfaces and clothing! I would caution you against wearing your nicest white blouse when opening a pomegranate, especially if you're new to the process.*

5 Fat Flush Herbs and Spices

Spice is the variety of life.

—JONNY BOWDEN, PhD, CNS

Herbs and spices flaunt Mother Nature in all her aromatic and healing glory. For thousands of years, people have utilized herbs and spices to flavor foods and treat illnesses: ginger for an upset tummy, cayenne for high blood pressure, cinnamon to lower blood sugar, garlic to ward off bacteria, nutmeg to warm digestion, and turmeric for just about everything including Alzheimer's and pain. Sadly, even with the wide array of spices available, black pepper remains the most popular seasoning among Americans!

I invite you to expand your use of herbs and spices to include a variety of Fat Flush flavors. For example, seasoning your foods with a bit of dill, parsley, coriander, or cumin goes a long way toward boosting the nutritional value of your meal and helps you steer clear of bloat-promoting salt and artificial additives.

What's the difference between an herb and a spice? An herb is an aromatic leaf, like parsley, while a spice stems from a pungent seed, root, or bark, such as cinnamon. Both types of seasonings offer a myriad of fat-flushing benefits, from urging the metabolism into high gear to erasing excess water weight.

Antioxidants, so abundant in herbs and spices, have become synonymous with good health because of their ability to neutralize harmful free radicals in the body. In addition, these Fat Flush seasonings aid the digestive process, support the liver, and help prevent disease. To achieve the greatest impact from seasonings, make use of the full range of Fat Flush herbs and spices. Avoid using any of the seasonings every day to prevent the development of food allergies. (People are prone to develop allergies to foods they eat all the time.)

The facts are indisputable. Herbs and spices transform the simplest meal by providing flavor and soul to your food. At the same time, they impart a host of nutritional rewards and are teeming with valuable health benefits. What more could you ask for from a *sprinkle of this* and a *dash of that*?

ANISE

Fat Flush Factors

Diuretic

What smells like licorice, tastes like licorice, but isn't licorice? It's anise, one of the oldest cultivated spices in the world. Native to the Middle East, anise has been used as a medicine since prehistoric times. The Romans used anise to thwart indigestion, prevent bad dreams, treat scorpion bites, and ward off the evil eye. In the sixteenth century, anise served as bait in mousetraps. These days, we have tastier uses for anise. It flavors cakes, cookies, and breads and enriches soups, stews, and seafood. From liqueurs to licorice candy, anise lends its distinctive flavor to a wide variety of food and drink.

Beyond the kitchen, anise is found in many commercial cough syrups and sore throat medications. In addition to adding flavor to these drugs, anise contains the chemicals creosol and alpha-pinene, which have been shown to loosen mucus in the bronchial tubes, thus making it easier to cough up. Studies have confirmed that anethole, the main active ingredient in anise, inhibits the growth of certain tumors, especially colon cancer. And scientists at the University of California found that anethole helps fight *Candida albicans*—those sugar-loving yeast microbes that can wreak havoc in our bodies.

Consuming anise can soothe a queasy stomach and boost antioxidant levels, and because it contains dianethole and photoanethole, which are chemically similar to estrogen, anise can even take the edge off perimenopausal symptoms.

Recommended Usage
Up to one teaspoon of anise seeds per week.

Just the Facts
• Licorice candy contains very little "licorice." Instead, most of its flavor comes from anise.
• Mexico is the world's largest producer of anise.
• Anise "perfumes" the artificial rabbit used in greyhound races.
• In medicine, anise oil masks the taste of bitter-tasting drugs.

Be a Fat Flush Cook

- For a refreshing taste, sprinkle a few anise seeds onto a salad or mix some into your salad dressing.
- When you're cooking cabbage, add anise seeds to produce a delightful flavor.
- Sprinkle a bit of ground anise in hot lemon water. Drink it first thing in the morning to give your digestive system a boost.
- Baked apples are delicious with ground anise seed sprinkled on top.
- Store anise in a cool, dry, dark place in tightly sealed containers. Anise may retain its flavor qualities and strength for up to three years.

IT'S BEEN SAID . . .

Once you get a spice in your home, you have it forever. Women never throw out spices. The Egyptians were buried with their spices. I know which one I'm taking with me when I go.

ERMA BOMBECK

Try steeping a teaspoon of anise seeds in hot water to make a Fat Flush-friendly tea. It makes a refreshing and elegant drink after dinner.

CINDY C., CALIFORNIA

CAYENNE

Fat Flush Factors
Energizer
Thermogenic

Cayenne has been used as both food and medicine in the tropical areas of South and Central America and Africa for more than 7,000 years. Related to both mild bell peppers and fiery chili peppers, cayenne bears no connection to black pepper. In fact, it was Spanish explorers who misnamed cayenne a pepper and began trading it around the world.

Cayenne does much more than create a tongue-tingling meal. It is loaded with vitamins C, B, A, and E and also contains calcium, phosphorus, and iron. One of the richest sources of vitamin E, cayenne helps keep the heart healthy and strong. And as its bright-red color suggests, it provides us with immune-boosting beta-carotene, one of the most important antioxidants in the body. Cayenne offers additional value as a painkiller (especially against the discomfort of arthritis), an antiseptic, and a digestive aid.

As most of us can attest, cayenne is a diaphoretic—a sweat-inducing spice. Its hotness comes from a high concentration of capsicum, a substance that has been firing up the circulation for centuries. It is capsicum that gives cayenne the power to get the blood pumping efficiently, stimulate the body's metabolic rate, and help clean fat out of the arteries. Cayenne adds a real kick to all your veggies, sauces, dips, and soups. I even like a pinch of this hot stuff in my smoothie.

A study at Oxford Polytechnic Institute proved that cayenne pepper stimulates the metabolism by about 20 percent and results in increased distribution of oxygen throughout the body.

Recommended Usage
Liberal use, to taste, every other day.

Just the Facts
• Capsicum, the colorless, heat-producing compound in cayenne, is also known as capsaicin. Amazingly, within the last few years, over 1,300 studies on capsicum have been published in medical journals.

- Because of its hot, burning flavor, cayenne takes its name from a Greek word meaning "to bite."
- People who break out in a sweat after eating cayenne are experiencing "gustatory perspiration."
- Dropping a pinch of cayenne into your gloves will keep your hands warm on a cold morning.
- You may see cayenne ranging in color from deep red to nearly orange.
- Cayenne is one of the few spices that are always purchased in ground form.

Boost the Benefits
- Cayenne pepper should be kept in a tightly sealed glass jar, away from direct sunlight. Stored in this way, it should keep up to one year.

Be a Fat Flush Cook
- Cayenne is sure to heat up any combination of mixed, steamed veggies.
- Give your herbal coffee a traditional Mexican flair by adding a tiny bit of cayenne pepper.
- Adding cayenne and lemon juice to cooked bitter greens, such as kale, really complements the flavor.
- Use cayenne in moderation. For example, for a recipe that serves four, start with just a dash or two. Increase the amount, dash by dash, until you have the heat level you desire.
- Because cayenne's heat intensifies when it's frozen, you may want to go easy when making a dish destined for the freezer.

THINK TWICE!
- *Keep cayenne away from your eyes and moist mucous membranes.*
- *When making smoothies, don't mistake your bottle of cayenne for cinnamon. This happened to one unlucky Fat Flusher who experienced a whole new taste sensation that morning!*

IT'S BEEN SAID . . .

I've banished my salt and pepper shakers. Instead, I keep a container of cayenne on the table so I can rev up my metabolism at most every meal.

JULIE T., WASHINGTON

CINNAMON

Fat Flush Factors

Blood Sugar Stabilizer
Thermogenic

Once considered a precious commodity, cinnamon boasts a long history as both a spice and a medicine. Cinnamon is actually tree bark and can be found in dried stick form or as a ground powder. True cinnamon comes from Ceylon and is difficult to find in U.S. stores. Tan in color, it offers a delicate aroma and a sweeter flavor than the more common, less expensive "cassia" cinnamon. If the cinnamon in your cupboard is mahogany red, it is cassia and was probably grown in Vietnam, China, Indonesia, or Central America.

Medieval physicians treated coughs, sore throats, and diarrhea with cinnamon. Europeans used cinnamon to preserve foods and to mask the stench and flavor of spoiling meats. And it turns out that they were on to something. Recent studies have confirmed cinnamon's ability to rid foods of dangerous bacteria. One study, conducted at Kansas State University, found that cinnamon destroyed *E. coli* bacteria in apple juice.

The healing powers of cinnamon's active ingredients (cinnamaldehyde, cinnamyl acetate, and cinnamyl alcohol) don't end there. Cinnamon has been well researched for its ability to prevent unwanted clumping of blood platelets. Cinnamon consumption can boost the metabolism and derail candida, the microorganism that causes yeast overgrowth in the body. The calcium and fiber content of cinnamon seems to improve intestinal health and protect against heart disease. And best of all, in both test-tube and animal studies, scientists at the U.S. Department of Agriculture have found that cinnamon makes cells more responsive to insulin. Clinical trials with humans are currently under way, but it appears that just a dash of cinnamon can help the body to metabolize glucose, keeping blood sugar levels in check.

I only recommend Ceylon cinnamon because most commercial cinnamons contain the liver-damaging ingredient coumarin that can be harmful to health when taken in excess. Cinnamon in general, however, is most helpful in controlling blood sugar levels so that insulin spikes are kept in check, and it can even reduce the glycemic impact of a meal by nearly 30 percent. As a delicious metabolism booster, cinnamon can rock desserts, lamb, coffee, tea, and smoothies.

Recommended Usage

One-half to one teaspoon every other day.

Just the Facts

• In the United States, consumption of cinnamon has jumped by 6.5 million pounds in the last decade.

• Most of the "cinnamon" sold across the United States is actually cassia (although it is labeled as cinnamon). Cinnamon and cassia are closely related, but cassia is stronger and less delicate in flavor. True cinnamon is readily available in other countries, including Mexico.

• Cinnamon sticks are known officially as "quills."

• If you consume cinnamon every day, your body may stop responding to its thermogenic properties.

• How can you tell if your cinnamon sticks are true cinnamon or cassia? True cinnamon quills curl up from one side, like a jellyroll, while cassia quills roll inward from both sides, like a scroll.

Boost the Benefits

• To ensure the best flavor and nutrition from your cinnamon, buy it in small quantities, because it becomes stale quickly, losing both flavor and aroma. Your best bet is to grind your own cinnamon from quills, using a spice or coffee grinder.

• Keep your cinnamon in a tightly sealed glass container in a cool, dark, and dry place. Ground cinnamon keeps for about six months, while cinnamon sticks stay fresh for about one year. To check for freshness, *smell* your cinnamon. Discard it if the aroma is no longer sweet.

• Foods that undergo radiation during their processing may form free radicals that are potentially harmful to humans. Look for organically grown cinnamon, because it has likely not been irradiated. Among other potentially harmful effects, irradiating cinnamon can reduce its vitamin C and carotenoid content.

Be a Fat Flush Cook

• To prevent the bitterness that comes with extended cooking, add ground cinnamon to your dish shortly before you serve it.

• Try a dash of cinnamon in spaghetti sauce, beef stew, or chili.

• Brighten the flavor of apple, peach, or pear slices with a sprinkle of cinnamon.

• Before broiling, season chicken breasts or lamb chops with some sweet-spicy cinnamon.

Fat Flush Fun

* To fill your home with the scent of cinnamon, simmer a quill or two in a pot of water. This is especially nice throughout the winter holidays.

IT'S BEEN SAID . . .

To give your stir-fry a Middle Eastern flair, simmer a cinnamon quill in a few tablespoons of broth until it unrolls; then add your other ingredients.

PATTY R., TEXAS

CLOVES

Fat Flush Factors

Thermogenic

Did you know that cloves are actually flower buds, picked and dried before they blossom? Shaped like nails, whole cloves are an easy spice to recognize and have been prized throughout the ages. In ancient China, people were required to freshen their mouths by chewing cloves prior to meeting the emperor, and in the Spice Islands, wars were fought over the right to grow and sell cloves. Today, Brazil, Indonesia, and Zanzibar all produce cloves, although the finest cloves are said to come from Madagascar.

Eugenol, the main component of cloves, has a long-standing reputation for killing bacteria and viruses. This explains why cloves have been valued throughout history as a food preservative, a wound disinfectant, and a toothache cure. Highly antiseptic, clove oil continues to be used in mouthwashes, medicines, and antacids.

As a Fat Flush food, cloves stimulate digestion, fire up the metabolism, and reduce intestinal bloating and gas. So keep this hot, slightly sweet spice handy. You can try whole cloves to give an intense "punch" to your food, or you can use ground cloves for a more subdued flavor.

Recommended Usage

An eighth to a quarter teaspoon two to three times per week.

Just the Facts

• Cloves serve as natural insect repellents for ants and other crawling insects.
• Cloves are the only spice that is smoked more than it is eaten. Indonesia uses half the world's supply of cloves to make "kretek" cigarettes. (The American Lung Association has declared that clove cigarettes are even more toxic than tobacco.)

Boost the Benefits

- Because of their high oil content, you need to keep cloves tightly covered, or they will lose flavor and turn rancid. Store this spice away from the light, in an airtight container.
- Look for whole cloves that are mahogany red, are slightly oily, and give off a pungent, sweet aroma. Avoid black or shriveled cloves; they are not fresh.
- Get rid of any ground clove that tastes bitter or harsh. It's too old.

Be a Fat Flush Cook

- Use cloves sparingly because the flavor continues to develop in a dish over time.
- Add cloves to tomato dishes or sprinkle them over cooked sweet potato.
- Do you make your own broth? Push a clove or two into an onion to give a distinctive flavor to chicken or vegetable broth.

IT'S BEEN SAID . . .

Several times a week, I add a pinch of cloves to my morning smoothie. It's especially good in a peach smoothie!

CAROL A., CALIFORNIA

CORIANDER

> ## Fat Flush Factors
> ### Blood Sugar Stabilizer

Coriander—is it an herb or a spice? How about *both*? The fresh minty sweet leaves are considered an herb and are sometimes called cilantro or Chinese parsley. The seeds, which look like tan peppercorns, are a fragrant spice and taste like a mixture of sweet orange peel and sage.

Coriander is probably one of the first herbs to be used by people, going back as far as 5000 BC. If you read *Tales of the Arabian Nights*, you'll see coriander mentioned as an aphrodisiac. In ancient China, eating coriander was a way to ensure immortality. Coriander holds the honor of being one of the first spices to arrive in America, and it sits high on the list of the healing spices.

Coriander is traditionally known as an "antidiabetic" plant. This claim has recently been confirmed. The *British Journal of Nutrition* published a study that found that when coriander was added to the diet of diabetic mice, it helped stimulate their secretion of insulin and lowered their blood sugar.

Currently, scientists are taking a look at coriander for its cholesterol-lowering effects. Researchers at a university in India fed coriander to rats that were on a high-fat, high-cholesterol diet. They found that coriander lowered levels of total and LDL cholesterol while actually increasing HDL levels. While further research is needed, there is no doubt that coriander packs a wallop as a Fat Flush food.

Recommended Usage
Up to one bunch per week.

Just the facts
- Coriander stalks are tender and have the same flavor as the leaves—so don't throw them out!
- Only a small amount of coriander is needed to flavor dishes, especially if you're using fresh coriander.

Boost the Benefits

- When buying fresh coriander, look for vibrantly deep-green leaves that are firm, crisp, and unspotted.
- Fresh coriander leaves are perishable and won't keep more than a few days. To maximize storage time, wrap the leaves in a moist cloth and refrigerate them in a loosely fitting plastic bag. If the roots are intact, store the bouquet of coriander in a glass of water and cover it loosely with a plastic bag.
- Bunched coriander can be frozen by simply wrapping it in foil before placing it in the freezer.
- To keep coriander seeds, either whole or ground, store them in a tightly sealed container away from light. Ground coriander keeps for about four months, while whole seeds stay fresh for at least one year.
- Wash and chop fresh coriander right before adding it to your dish since the aroma of coriander intensifies immediately after being cut. To clean your coriander, place it in a bowl of cold water and swish it around with your hands. Repeat this process with clean water until no dirt remains in the bowl.
- To intensify the flavor of whole coriander seeds, toast them in a dry, nonstick frying pan before you grind them.

Be a Fat Flush Cook

- To enjoy the peak flavor of fresh coriander leaves, add them to your dish during the last few moments of cooking.
- Season fish with lemon juice, coriander, and mustard. Then broil for a delectable flavor.
- Stir-fry some spinach, fresh garlic, and coriander seeds. Season with ginger and cumin, and you've got a side dish that's jam packed with nutrients.
- Substitute fresh coriander for parsley or chervil in most any recipe.
- Toss fresh coriander leaves with salad greens for an added zing.

IT'S BEEN SAID . . .

I put coriander seeds in a pepper mill and keep it on the dinner table to give many of my Fat Flush meals an extra boost of flavor.

CARYL P., NORTH CAROLINA

CUMIN

Fat Flush Factors
Detoxifier

An ordinary-looking seed, cumin packs a punch when it comes to both flavor and health benefits. Cumin has a distinctive taste, slightly bitter and peppery with a hint of citrus, which it lends to a wide array of Mexican, Indian, and Middle Eastern dishes. In the kitchens of ancient Greece and Rome, cumin served as a replacement for black pepper, which was expensive and hard to come by. During the Middle Ages, Europeans recognized cumin as a symbol of love and fidelity. Wives baked loaves of cumin bread to give to their husbands as they headed off to war.

Today, cumin is experiencing a comeback, as more people come to appreciate its culinary and therapeutic properties. Cumin seed is high in protein, potassium, iron, and thiamine. Researchers are finding that cumin stimulates the secretion of pancreatic enzymes, thereby aiding digestion and absorption of nutrients. Because of its ability to scavenge for free radicals, cumin enhances the detoxification process in the liver. And two of cumin's active ingredients, carevol and limonene, have been shown to be powerful cancer fighters.

Whether you select the black or yellow-brown variety, be sure to add a healthy dose of cumin to your diet. Your liver will thank you.

This peppery biblical spice is a wonderful taste enhancer and catalyst for weight loss. The latest research out of the Middle East, where cumin is popularly consumed, shows that one teaspoon of this spice boosts weight loss by 50 percent, most likely due to its ability to raise body temperature, thereby heating up metabolism. This is one great spice for hummus, beans, chili, and any variation of a Mexican food dish.

Recommended Usage

Liberal use, to taste, every other day.

Just the Facts

- Cumin ranks as one of the most popular spices in the world, second only to black pepper.
- Cumin "seeds" are actually the small dried fruits of the cumin plant.

- Cumin is the essential ingredient in chili powder.

Boost the Benefits

- Whether whole or ground, cumin seeds should be stored in tightly sealed glass containers in a cool, dry place. Ground cumin keeps for about six months, while the whole seeds stay fresh for up to one year.
- Whenever possible, buy whole cumin seeds instead of powder since ground cumin loses its flavor more quickly than the seeds. You can easily grind your own cumin with a mortar and pestle.
- To bring out their full aroma and flavor, lightly roast whole cumin seeds before using them in a recipe.
- When making a dish that needs to simmer for a long time, consider using *whole* cumin seeds. Ground cumin can quickly lose its strength and become bitter.

Be a Fat Flush Cook

- Add cumin to beef to give a new twist to pot roast or stew recipes.
- Flavor lamb brochettes or kebabs with cumin and then grill.
- Season steamed vegetables with cumin to give them a North African flair.

IT'S BEEN SAID . . .

On those days when I'm not planning a meal with cumin, I make myself a cup of warming cumin tea by boiling the seeds in water and then letting them steep for 8 to 10 minutes.

DONNA F., PENNSYLVANIA

DANDELION

Fat Flush Factors
Blood Sugar Stabilizer
Detoxifier
Diuretic
Thermogenic

Before you go yanking out those pesky dandelions and tossing them into the compost pile, you may want to check out their health benefits. What many folks consider irritating weeds are actually secret stockpiles of phytonutrients with amazing health benefits. Every part of the dandelion plant has nutritional gifts to bear, including cancer preventatives—from the tips of their leaves to the ends of their seemingly endless roots.

Dandelions belong to one of the largest plant families, the sunflower family (Asteraceae), which also includes daisies and thistles. They have been used medicinally as far back as the tenth century in the Middle East for everything from anemia to scurvy, skin problems, blood disorders, and depression.

At the present time, Green Med Info's database for dandelions lists 47 scientific abstracts cataloging the plant's evidence-based health benefits, with the strongest studies pointing toward anti-inflammatory and antioxidant properties that affect just about every system in your body. Dandelions' anti-inflammatory properties make them useful for relieving muscle and joint aches, soothing eczema, and reducing postinjury redness and swelling. Dandelions offer support to your immune system, such as helping combat antibiotic-resistant infections.

Underlying these benefits is a nutritional bounty that includes vitamin C, B vitamins, beta-carotene, potassium, iron, calcium, magnesium, manganese, copper, zinc, phosphorus, and even some vitamin D. Dandelion greens provide a staggering 535 percent of the recommended daily amount for vitamin K (K1, not K2). They are rich in fiber and boast more protein than spinach.

These superweeds act as both diuretic and laxative. They help your kidneys flush out waste by ramping up urine production, as well as increasing the activity of your digestive tract—especially fat digestion. Dandelions boost your bile production, keeping it thin and smooth flowing, which reduces gallstones. Dandelion has also been shown to help with nausea, loss of appetite, gas, and bloating. Dandelion promotes detox by reducing inflammation in your liver and gallbladder, promoting electrolyte balance and good hydration, and helping your liver filter out toxins, and it's even been used to treat jaundice.

But wait—there's more! Dandelions have anti-obesity properties and can lower your risk for type 2 diabetes, which is epidemic today. They stabilize blood sugar by stimulating your pancreas to produce more insulin, as well as lowering your blood pressure and working magic on your cholesterol and other lipids.

As a huge bonus, your cup of dandelion tea may keep you out of the oncologist's office. Dandelion root was found to cause melanoma cells to self-destruct (apoptosis)—even drug-resistant ones. Additionally, in 2011 researchers discovered that dandelion root tea may contain a "kill switch" for leukemia cells. Other studies have shown dandelion to exert similar effects against cancers of the breast and prostate.

Recommended Usage

- All parts of the dandelion are safe to eat. Leaves, roots, stems, and flowers can be consumed raw, as part of a salad, or cooked as you would any other greens (steamed or sautéed). Cooking, as well as adding some lemon juice, helps minimize dandelion's somewhat bitter flavor.
- Dandelion roots, stems, and flowers can be brewed into a delicious antioxidant-rich tea. The root is classically used for tea, but if roasted first, you get "dandelion coffee." Dandelion tea is useful for enhancing digestion before or after a meal and for treating indigestion after a fatty meal.

Just the Facts

- Dandelions are thought to have evolved about 30 million years ago in Eurasia. Their name is derived from the French words *dent de lion*, meaning "lion's tooth." Two species grow worldwide: *Taraxacum officinale* and *T. erythrospermum*.
- Dandelions attract pollinators and release ethylene gas, which helps fruit ripen.
- Dandelions have an underground taproot that can grow to a whopping 15 feet! This taproot adds minerals and nitrogen to the soil, as well as bringing nutrients upward to feed more shallowly rooted plants.
- The milky white sap you get on your fingers when you break a dandelion stem has germicidal, insecticidal, and fungicidal properties; it can be used to relieve itching related to eczema, psoriasis, ringworm, or insect bites.

- Dandelions may have the longest flowering season of any plant. Their blossoms were historically used to treat warts, blisters, and other skin afflictions.

Boost the Benefits

- Dandelion parts will stay fresh in your fridge for about a week, and wrapping them in a damp paper towel may extend freshness. The good news is, if your dandelion greens are past their prime, there are probably *more* where those came from!

Fat Flush in Action

- How to make dandelion tea or coffee: Chop clean dandelion roots by hand or in a food processor. For tea, steep root pieces in boiling water for 10 to 30 minutes; then strain. For a nutritious caffeine-free coffee alternative, arrange chopped roots on a baking sheet and roast for two hours in a 300 degree oven before steeping.

THINK TWICE!

- *Make sure to collect your dandelions from areas not sprayed with herbicides.*
- *Some people have allergic reactions to dandelion. If you are allergic to ragweed or related plants (daisies, chrysanthemums, marigolds, yarrow, daisy, chamomile, etc.), be very cautious about trying dandelion.*
- *Dandelion has some potential drug interactions. If you take dandelion along with a drug (such as several types of antibiotics), it may reduce the drug's absorption, thereby decreasing effectiveness. Dandelion may also affect certain medications by way of its diuretic properties, altering urinary clearance and affecting your blood levels. Two examples are lithium and potassium. Dandelion may also decrease how quickly your liver breaks down and clears certain drugs out of your body.*

Fat Flush Fun

- Dandelion is the only flower that represents all three celestial bodies—the sun, the moon, and the stars. The yellow flower is said to represent the sun, the puff ball signifies the moon, and the dispersing seeds represent the stars.

- Dandelion roots may be used to make dandelion beer.
- For your health and the health of the planet, consider ditching chemical herbicides, along with your need for the perfectly "manicured" grass lawn. Every year, Americans spend millions of dollars on toxic lawn chemicals and use 30 percent of the country's water supply to keep their lawns green. What about a vegetable garden instead? You could be the first one on your block to sport a dedicated dandelion patch.

IT'S BEEN SAID . . .

Only the wind knows where it will carry our dandelion souls.

A. R. ASHER

When you look at a field of dandelions, you can see either a hundred weeds or a thousand wishes.

UNKNOWN

DILL

Fat Flush Factors
Diuretic

Dill offers double the pleasure—and Fat Flush power—since *both* its leaves and seeds may be used as a seasoning. Dill's fern-like, green leaves are delicate and have a soft, sweet taste. Dried dill seeds are light-brown ovals with a sweet, citrusy flavor.

One of the favorite herbs in ancient Greece and Rome, dill was considered good luck and was often placed in a baby's cradle or over a door jamb for protection. Ancient soldiers applied roasted dill seeds to their wounds to encourage healing and help prevent infection. Today, we know those soldiers were on to something. Current research has confirmed that dill prevents bacterial overgrowth.

In addition to serving as a natural diuretic, dillweed contains a substance called carvone, which aids and calms digestion by relieving intestinal gas. This probably explains why, in early America, children were given dill seeds to calm them during lengthy church services. It also explains why I promote the frequent use of dill. The digestive tract works less efficiently as we age, and consuming dill gives it a welcomed boost.

As an added bonus, the active ingredients in dill qualify it as a "chemoprotective" food that helps neutralize certain carcinogens, such as the benzopyrenes found in cigarette smoke, charcoal grill smoke, and the smoke produced by trash incinerators. So use dill liberally to detox your body and delight your taste buds.

Recommended Usage
Two teaspoons per week.

Just the Facts
- It takes a tablespoon of chopped fresh dill to equal one teaspoon of dried dillweed.
- An ounce of dill seeds contains more than 10,000 tiny seeds.
- One tablespoon of dill seed contains as much calcium as a cup of milk. Dill is also a good source of fiber, iron, and magnesium.

Boost the Benefits

- When shopping for fresh dill, look for feathery green leaves. Don't worry if the leaves appear slightly wilted, because they usually droop very quickly after being picked.
- Store fresh dill in the refrigerator either wrapped in a damp paper towel or placed with its stems upright in a container of water—like a bouquet of flowers. Since it is very fragile, dill keeps fresh for only a few days, even if stored properly.
- Forget using a knife and cutting board. Snip fresh dill with scissors to mince the delicate leaves.
- Your best bet for long-term storage is to freeze dill leaves. To use the frozen leaves, just snip off what you need and drop the rest back in the freezer. (Dill tends to darken a bit in the freezer, but it keeps nicely for several months.)
- For handy access when making soups, stews, or stir-fries, freeze dill leaves in ice-cube trays covered with broth. Then pop out just as many cubes as you need.
- Keep dried dill seeds in a tightly sealed glass container. If you keep the container in a cool, dry, dark place, the dill seeds will stay fresh for about six months.
- There is no comparison between the flavor of fresh dill and dried dill-weed. Use fresh for the most intense flavor. If you must use dried, do so with a generous hand.

Fat Flush Fun

- Rumor has it that if you sprinkle some fresh dill leaves in your bath-water, you will be irresistible to your lover!

Be a Fat Flush Cook

- The longer that dillweed is cooked, the more the flavor diminishes. Add it at the last minute to achieve full flavor and aroma.
- Combine dillweed with plain yogurt and chopped cucumber for a delicious cooling dip or tangy seafood sauce.
- When broiling lamb chops or steak, sprinkle chopped fresh dill on the meat during the last five minutes.
- Is fish on the menu? The flavor of dill enhances most fish very well, especially salmon and trout.
- Since dill seeds are known for soothing the stomach after a meal, put some seeds in a small dish and pass them around the dinner table for everyone to enjoy.

DRIED MUSTARD

Fat Flush Factors
Thermogenic

Can you guess what mustard and broccoli have in common? They are both members of the cruciferous family of vegetables. While there are about 40 different types of mustard plants, we get seeds from three main varieties: black, white, and brown mustard. For the most pungent flavor, look for *black* mustard seeds. *White* mustard seeds are the mildest and are used to make American yellow mustard. Dijon mustard contains the flavorful, dark-yellow seeds of the *brown* mustard plant.

At first, mustard was considered a medicine rather than a food. In the sixth century BC, the Greek scientist Pythagoras used mustard to take the bite out of scorpion stings. One hundred years later, Hippocrates treated patients with mustard medicines and poultices. Around the globe, people in every culture continued to find uses for mustard. German folklore encouraged brides who wanted to rule the roost to sew mustard seeds into the hem of their wedding dresses, while from Denmark to India mustard was sprinkled around the outside of homes to ward off evil spirits. It was the early Romans who ground mustard seeds and mixed them with wine into a paste similar to the prepared mustards of today.

Mustard seeds contain ample amounts of phytonutrients, including isothiocyanates. The isothiocyanates in mustard seeds have been the focus of many cancer-related studies and have been shown to inhibit the growth of existing cancer cells, especially in gastrointestinal tumors.

Mustard seeds provide selenium, magnesium, monounsaturated fats, and phosphorous. And they are a good source of iron, calcium, zinc, and manganese. Best of all, mustard helps flush fat by revving your metabolism. In a study conducted at the Oxford Polytechnic Institute in England, scientists found that spicy foods, especially mustard, spiked metabolic rates by 25 percent. By adding mustard to a meal, participants burned off at least 45 extra calories during the next three hours. So skip sugar-filled ketchup and stock up on dried mustard instead. Your waistline will thank you.

Mustard is a must in my kitchen. In the dried, powdered state or as a prepared mustard spread, it not only gives a burst of tangy spiciness, but helps flush fat by kicking metabolism into high gear. Study data from the Oxford Polytechnic Institute shows that mustard spikes metabolic rates by 25 percent. By adding mustard to a meal, participants burned at least 45 extra calories during the next three hours. Try just a pinch of dried mustard in your homemade salad dressings, mayo, and pickles. I really love it on my deviled eggs.

Recommended Usage

Liberal use, to taste, every other day.

Just the Facts

- Dry mustard contains at least twice the flavor zip of prepared mustard.
- The Fat Flush spice turmeric is what gives most American mustards their bright-yellow color.
- In the United States, pepper is the only spice consumed more often than mustard. And around the world, people eat over 700 million pounds of mustard every year.
- One teaspoon of dried mustard equals one tablespoon of prepared mustard.

Boost the Benefits

- When you mix dried mustard powder with cold water, a chemical reaction occurs between two enzymes that enhances the pungency and heat of the mustard. To stop the enzymatic process—and turn *down* the heat—you can add some very hot water or a bit of apple cider vinegar. Or just give it time. The mixture will reach its peak in fire and flavor after about 15 minutes and will quickly decline from that point on.
- Store whole mustard seeds in airtight containers in a cool, dry place for up to one year. Ground and powdered mustard stays fresh for up to six months.

Fat Flush Fun

- Try this tip during cold weather: sprinkle dry mustard inside your shoes to prevent cold feet and frostbite.
- Color your world yellow. Use mustard powder as a fertilizer—you'll get brighter-colored daffodils.

Be a Fat Flush Cook

- You may purchase mustard seeds either whole (and grind them yourself) or as a ground powder.
- For a tangy fat-flushing meal, dredge chicken breasts in "homemade" mustard and bake. Or use your mustard mixture as a dip for grilled chicken breast, fruits, and vegetables.
- Be creative with ground mustard, but go easy and taste along the way. You can always add more mustard, but there is no "cure" for overdoing it.

THINK TWICE!

- *Mustard seeds contain goitrogens, naturally occurring substances that can interfere with the functioning of the thyroid gland. If you have been diagnosed with a thyroid disorder, you may want to avoid ground mustard seeds.*
- *Easy does it when you're making your own mustard. Depending on the mustard powder, it's possible to make a mixture that actually burns or blisters your skin.*
- *Mustard contains sulfur, so steer clear if you have an allergy to sulfur.*

IT'S BEEN SAID . . .

My family loves Ann Louise's basic fat-flushing salad dressing as much as I do. Just mix equal parts flax oil and apple cider vinegar. Add dried mustard, fresh garlic, and minced dill to taste.

CANDY C., KENTUCKY

Mustard's no good without roast beef.

CHICO MARX, MONKEY BUSINESS

FENNEL SEED

Fat Flush Factors
Diuretic

Looking like tiny watermelons, greenish-gray fennel seeds give foods a subtle, sweet, licorice-like flavor. Yet fennel's reputation through the ages has been as a digestive soother. These unassuming little seeds can calm an acidic stomach, ease irritable bowel syndrome, and alleviate gas pains. As an added bonus, fennel relieves bloating by acting as a natural diuretic. How can this herb, which the Chinese used as a remedy for snakebites and scorpion stings, have such a soothing effect on the body? It appears that fennel relaxes smooth muscles in the body, including the lining of the digestive and urinary tracts.

Recent research suggests that anethole, the active ingredient in fennel, has an estrogen-like activity, making it a potential remedy for the symptoms of perimenopause. Anethole may also support the liver by encouraging the regeneration of liver cells, although more research is necessary to confirm this.

So whether you reach for fennel to season your food or chew a few seeds to settle your stomach after a big meal, you'll reap the benefits of this aromatic herb.

Recommended Usage

A maximum of one teaspoon of fennel seeds every other day. (The stems and the fronds may be eaten freely.)

Just the Facts

- Fennel comes from the Greek word for "marathon" because an ancient battle between the Greeks and the Persians was fought at Marathon on a field of fennel.
- Bulb fennel is a vegetable that resembles a plump celery plant.

Boost the Benefits

- To purchase good-quality fennel, look for seeds that are either yellow or greenish brown and that taste and smell a bit like licorice.
- Toasting fennel seeds enhances their flavor.

Be a Fat Flush Cook

- Typically used to complement fish, fennel is also found in a variety of Italian dishes.
- Sprinkle fennel and garlic on broiled lamb chops for a fabulous flavor.
- Add fennel to your favorite meatloaf recipe, sprinkle it over an apple before baking, or use a few seeds to season your next omelet.
- Fennel and fish are made for each other. Try adding some fennel seeds to the basting juices during cooking.

THINK TWICE!

- *If you have a history of an estrogen-dependent cancer, avoid fennel in significant quantities until more research is completed on fennel's estrogenic activity.*
- *Because it closely resembles poison hemlock, don't pick fennel in the wild unless you are an experienced herb harvester. Instead, rely on the fennel found at your local grocery.*

IT'S BEEN SAID . . .

To make one slender, take fennel, seethe it in water and drink it first and last, and it shall swaze either him or her.

THE GOOD HOUSEWIFE'S JEWELL, *1585*

For a terrific Fat Flush entrée, season a salmon steak with fennel, lemon juice, and a hint of garlic. Bake or broil and enjoy!

MAUREEN D., MARYLAND

GARLIC

Fat Flush Factors
Blood Sugar Stabilizer
Cholesterol Zapper
Detoxifier
Diuretic
Energizer

What would you expect to pay for a substance that can fight cancer, AIDS, and heart disease, lower both cholesterol and blood pressure by 10 percent, and serve as a natural antibiotic and antifungal medication? Put your calculators away. Garlic does all this and much more—for about 15 cents per clove. Mother Nature gave us the gift of garlic—a Fat Flush food that has been utilized as both food and medicine for over 5,000 years.

The health benefits of garlic are noted in both the Bible and the Talmud, and an Egyptian papyrus from 1500 BC recommends garlic as a treatment for a variety of ailments—from dog bites to bladder infections. Today, garlic is being heavily researched, and we have learned that it serves as a diuretic, a stimulant, and a sweat promoter. It stimulates the metabolism, stabilizes blood sugar levels, and eliminates toxins from the body.

Garlic contains a wide range of trace minerals, including copper, iron, zinc, magnesium, germanium, and especially selenium. In addition, garlic contains sulfur compounds, vitamins A and C, fiber, and various amino acids. In all, garlic provides more than 100 biologically useful chemicals. The active component of garlic is a sulfur compound known as allicin. This compound is generated only when a garlic clove is broken, and it is what gives raw, cut garlic its distinctive odor and pungent taste. Allicin also gives garlic its powerful Fat Flush punch. At least 12 studies have confirmed that allicin clears cholesterol from the blood. The largest study, conducted by German researchers on 261 participants, reported that total cholesterol levels dropped by 12 percent in 12 weeks in the group treated with garlic.

Recommended Usage
Two to six garlic cloves every other day.

Just the Facts

- One clove of garlic that's been pushed through a garlic press is 10 times stronger than one clove minced fine with a sharp knife.
- Chewing caraway seeds, fennel seeds, or fresh parsley after eating garlic helps freshen your breath.
- If you plant an individual garlic clove, it will reproduce an entire bulb in about nine months.

Boost the Benefits

- When you're shopping for garlic, look for plump, firm bulbs with plenty of dry, unbroken skin. Heads that show signs of sprouting are past their prime and were probably not dried properly. Garlic that is very old will crumble when it is gently squeezed.
- Store your garlic in a cool, dark, well-ventilated area, away from potatoes and onions. Do not refrigerate or keep in plastic containers. If stored in a damp, warm environment, garlic will sprout or become moldy.
- Unbroken garlic bulbs will keep for up to three months. Individual cloves stay fresh for about one week.
- To ensure proper digestion of garlic, make sure you remove the green "germ" in the middle of the clove.

Fat Flush Fun

- Don't try this at home! A famous French chef claims his success comes from chewing a small clove of garlic and then breathing gently on the salad before serving it.

Be a Fat Flush Cook

- To loosen garlic skin, place a clove on a cutting board and cover it with the flat side of a wide knife. Rap the blade sharply with your fist. Don't apply too much pressure, because the clove can easily be smashed.
- With garlic, the finer the chop, the stronger the taste. To lightly "perfume" your food with a mild garlic flavor, use whole, unbroken garlic cloves. Thin slices will provide more than a hint of garlic. For a fuller flavor, mince the garlic. And for an in-your-face garlic taste, crush the cloves to a pulp.

THINK TWICE!

- People who have bleeding disorders or who take anticoagulant medication should consult a doctor before using a garlic supplement or consuming large amounts of garlic.
- Stored at room temperature, garlic-in-oil mixtures provide perfect conditions for producing botulism toxin (low acidity, no free oxygen in the oil, and warm temperatures). Do not store raw or roasted garlic in oil at room temperature. You may store the mixture in the refrigerator for up to one week.

IT'S BEEN SAID . . .

A nickel will get you on the subway, but garlic will get you a seat.

OLD NEW YORK YIDDISH SAYING

I like to rub some crushed garlic on the inside of my salad bowl before adding the salad ingredients.

MICHELLE F., INDIANA

GINGER

> ## Fat Flush Factors
>
> Cholesterol Zapper
> Energizer
> Detoxifier

More than 5,000 years ago, people in ancient China and India regarded ginger as a "universal medicine." Today, ginger can be found in more than half of traditional herbal remedies. Throughout its long history, ginger has been used as a remedy for at least 40 conditions, as diverse as diarrhea, dizziness, menstrual cramps, and mumps.

Highly concentrated with active substances, including powerful antioxidants called "gingerols," ginger boasts a number of fat-flushing benefits. It revs circulation and promotes healthy sweating, encouraging detoxification of the body. Ginger supports liver function, clears up clogged arteries, and lowers serum cholesterol levels by nearly 30 percent. It contains compounds that resemble our digestive enzymes, assisting us to digest protein-rich meals more easily. And according to an Australian study published in the *Journal of Obesity*, ginger raises body temperature and assists the body to burn 20 percent more calories.

While hardly glamorous looking, with its knobby, gnarled appearance, ginger is a versatile and delicious Fat Flush food. The underground ginger stem, or rhizome, is a clump of flattish hand-like shapes ranging in color from pale greenish yellow to ivory. The aroma is pungent, and the flavor is peppery and slightly sweet.

Recommended Usage

At least a quarter-inch slice of fresh ginger every other day.

Just the Facts

- Ginger grows in many tropical areas including southern China, Japan, West Africa, and the Caribbean islands. Jamaican ginger is considered to be the best of all.
- Ginger is generally available in two forms, either young or mature. Most supermarkets carry mature ginger, which has a tough skin that

must be peeled. Young ginger, usually found only in Asian markets, does not require peeling.

• Ginger is a good source of calcium, phosphorus, iron, potassium, and vitamin A.

• Powdered ginger mixed with a bit of sea salt makes an excellent toothpaste, helping to strengthen gums and prevent bad breath.

Boost the Benefits

• Look for firm, plump "fingers" of fresh ginger, with clean, smooth skin. The smaller fingers tend to have the strongest flavor.

• When ginger is fresh, the flesh is pale yellow and very juicy. As it ages, it dries out and becomes fibrous, so avoid ginger that has become discolored, wrinkled, or moldy.

• The new little sprouts that appear on the sides of a gingerroot offer a delicate flavor, so don't be afraid to use them.

• Whenever possible, choose fresh ginger over dried, because fresh ginger tastes better *and* provides higher levels of gingerol.

• Fresh ginger can be stored in the refrigerator for up to three weeks if it is left unpeeled. Stored unpeeled in the freezer, it will keep for up to six months.

• Keep dried ginger powder in a tightly sealed glass container in a cool, dark, and dry place. Better yet, store it in the refrigerator to extend its shelf life to at least one year.

Be a Fat Flush Cook

• To substitute fresh ginger for ground ginger in your recipes, use a one-inch piece of freshly grated gingerroot for every quarter teaspoon of ground ginger.

• To peel ginger, use the edge of a spoon to scrape the skin off. It should almost roll off—without wasting any of the flesh.

• Spice up cranberry juice with some freshly grated ginger.

• Grate some fresh ginger onto your Fat Flush sweet potatoes.

• To create a flavor base for a stir-fry, mince some fresh ginger and sauté it in broth with some garlic.

• Add grated ginger and ground flax seed to apples and bake for a yummy dessert.

• Give zip to a rainbow of sautéed vegetables by adding freshly minced ginger.

THINK TWICE!

* Did you know that ginger is a blood thinner? So if you are taking a prescription blood thinner, avoid ingesting ginger.

IT'S BEEN SAID . . .

Don't be afraid to spice up that a.m. smoothie. A big chunk of fresh ginger (about a square inch) will give it a bit of zing and help your metabolism.

MARY D., FLORIDA

An I had but one penny in the world, thou should'st have it to buy gingerbread.

WILLIAM SHAKESPEARE, LOVE'S LABOURS LOST

PARSLEY

Fat Flush Factors
Diuretic

Parsley is the most widely used herb in the United States; yet every year, tons of this green garnish end up in the garbage. You should think twice about ignoring those decorative sprigs, because parsley contains more beta-carotene than carrots, more vitamin C than oranges, more calcium than a cup of milk, and twice as much iron as spinach. It is also a good source of niacin, vitamin B6, folate, phosphorus, zinc, copper, and fiber.

Through the ages, parsley has been used as a blood purifier and a natural diuretic. Its ability to rid the body of excess water and toxins makes it a shoo-in as a Fat Flush food. Parsley's high nutritional value gives it the power to promote good digestion, nourish the liver, and strengthen the adrenal glands. In addition, parsley contains the essential oil apiole, which helps stimulate the kidneys and fight water retention. By making parsley part of your regular diet, you can lower your heart rate, reduce your blood pressure, and banish monthly bloat. As an added benefit, the high chlorophyll content in parsley will keep your breath fresh and sweet.

Recommended Usage

One bunch of fresh parsley per week.

Just the Facts

- The Greeks crowned the victors of ancient games with parsley wreaths.
- In the Hebrew celebration of Passover, parsley symbolizes spring and rebirth.
- While there are more than 30 varieties of parsley, curly-leaf parsley, a common garnish, is the most popular, and Italian, or flat-leaf, parsley offers the best flavor for cooking.
- It takes 12 pounds of fresh parsley to make 1 pound of dried; yet dried parsley has only *half* the taste and minerals of fresh parsley.

Boost the Benefits

• Select healthy, fresh-looking bunches with bright-green, crisp leaves.
• Keep parsley fresh by moistening a paper towel and wrapping it around the parsley bunch. Place in a plastic bag and store it in the refrigerator for up to one week.
• You can freshen slightly wilted leaves by standing the stems in cold water. However, this causes some loss of vitamin C.
• Like many other herbs, fresh parsley can be frozen. Wash the parsley and pat it dry. After chopping it, put the parsley in a plastic bag and toss it in the freezer. When you're ready to cook it, just take out what you need. It will thaw almost immediately.
• Remember that cooking parsley for a long time takes away from its flavor and nutrient value, so add it toward the end of cooking.
• To intensify the flavor of *any* dried herb, sprinkle it over fresh parsley leaves before you chop them.

Be a Fat Flush Cook

• To reap the benefits of parsley, use it fresh by tossing a handful into your salad or sprinkling minced leaves over cooked foods.
• Mix some freshly minced parsley and garlic into flaxseed oil for a savory, yet simple, topping for steamed vegetables.
• Parsley enriches the flavor of any broth. Stir some parsley leaves—and stems—into homemade or canned broth.
• If you add too much garlic to a broth or soup, you can remove some by inserting parsley leaves into a tea infuser and placing the infuser in the broth. The parsley attracts the garlic.

IT'S BEEN SAID . . .

You might want to try drying your own parsley. I spread freshly gathered parsley on a piece of parchment paper and place in a 200 degree oven with the door cracked open. As soon as the parsley is dry, I crush it and put it in a bottle with a cork stopper. The parsley stays green and flavorful this way.

SANDY S., MASSACHUSETTS

TURMERIC

Fat Flush Factors

Blood Sugar Stabilizer
Cholesterol Zapper
Detoxifier
Thermogenic

It would take an entire book to cover the health benefits of turmeric. Thermogenesis, detoxification, diabetes, depression, kidney health, cancer, pain and inflammation, cardiovascular disease, cognitive function—I wonder if there's any condition this gold mine doesn't help. If so, we probably just haven't discovered it yet. It's arguably the most powerful herb on the planet and the perfect partner for Fat Flushers.

There are more than 9,000 peer-reviewed studies on PubMed about the benefits of turmeric and its primary active compound, curcumin. Turmeric facilitates healing in more than 800 different conditions by at least 150 therapeutic actions and has the ability to modulate more than 700 genes. In fact, this superroot packs so much punch that when compared with conventional medication, its benefits match or outperform many drugs and do so with far fewer adverse reactions. What follows are only the highlights.

Turmeric root is the spice most frequently used in curries, particularly yellow curries, and an excellent source of iron, manganese, vitamin B6, copper, potassium, and dietary fiber. What makes turmeric root really special is a particular group of polyphenols called curcuminoids (curcumin, bisdemethoxycurcumin, and demethoxycurcumin), as well as a few volatile oils (tumerone, atlantone, and zingiberone), which all offer unique health benefits. Turmeric's most extensively studied compound, curcumin, typically accounts for about 2 to 5 percent of the root weight.

For starters, turmeric helps your liver filter out toxins, as well as flushing out the ones trapped in body fat. Curcumin can actually attach itself to capsaicin receptors to boost thermogenesis. More than one study shows curcumin's ability to inhibit fat genesis, reducing overall body fat and supporting weight loss.

This golden root has fabulous benefits for your heart, improving blood pressure and regulating blood fat levels after meals. Curcumin is equal to or more effective than diabetes medications in reducing inflammation and oxidative stress. One study showed curcumin to be 400 to

100,000 times more potent than metformin (a common diabetes drug) for improving insulin sensitivity. Curcumin also outperforms many anticoagulant drugs among those at high risk for blood clots.

As an anti-inflammatory and pain treatment, turmeric blows away the competition. Curcumin is arguably one of the most potent anti-inflammatory compounds in the world, which is big news because most of our chronic diseases today—cancer, cognitive decline, ulcerative colitis, arthritis, heart disease, and others—result from inflammation. In one study, curcumin worked significantly better than diclofenac sodium (a drug for rheumatoid arthritis), without the adverse effects of the drug. A 2015 meta-analysis found curcumin to be a safe and effective pain intervention warranting further study.

Turmeric offers benefits to those suffering from Crohn's disease, ulcerative colitis, inflammatory bowel disease (IBD), and a number of other digestive problems. This is thought to be related to how it changes cell signaling and decreases production of pro-inflammatory cytokines.

For example, curcumin helps heal the gut and supports the growth of beneficial microflora in those with IBD, without the side effects of corticosteroids. For many IBD sufferers, corticosteroids reduce pain but tear up the intestinal lining over time, making symptoms worse. Curcumin has also been found useful against *H. pylori* infections including gastritis, peptic ulcer, and stomach cancer, as well as exhibiting other antimicrobial actions. Speaking of cancer, turmeric is unique in that it appears to exhibit anticancer activity against nearly all forms of cancer (breast, skin, stomach, liver, and many others), preventing their growth and spread. Chemotherapy is also more effective when combined with turmeric.

Curcumin has been found to have unique brain benefits for improving mood and cognitive function and reducing your risk for stroke and neurodegenerative disease. Turmeric's compound tumerone helps repair stem cells in the brain, speeding stroke recovery and slowing down the progression of dementia. When turmeric was compared with fluoxetine (Prozac) for major depressive disorder, it was found equally effective but with fewer side effects. As you can see, turmeric is unparalleled in its health-boosting power, so if you incorporate it into your daily diet, every cell in your body will be thanking you!

Recommended Usage

- The dose of turmeric you need to receive health benefits is not huge— as little as one-fiftieth of a teaspoon daily over a period of months has been shown to produce positive benefits.
- Adding turmeric to your green drinks adds a little extra flavor and a lot of nutritional kick.

- Add turmeric to your egg salad or deviled eggs to boost their nutritional value and intensify their color.
- Turmeric is fabulous with lentils, quinoa, and other high-nutrition grains.
- Turmeric and cauliflower are natural mates! Cut cauliflower florets in half and sauté with a generous spoonful of turmeric for five minutes. Once off the heat, toss with flax oil, a dash of sea salt, and pepper to taste.

Just the Facts

- Turmeric is not the same as curry. Curry is the general term for any number of spice blends (especially Indian), many of which have turmeric as one component.
- Turmeric comes from the root of the *Curcuma longa* plant and, along with ginger and cardamom, belongs to the Zingiberaceae family.
- Turmeric root is native to India and Southeast Asia, with medical use dating back thousands of years, in the Ayurvedic tradition.
- About 800,000 tons of turmeric is produced each year worldwide, with more than 75 percent originating in India.

Boost the Benefits

- Curcumin stimulates production of DHA (docosahexaenoic acid) from ALA (alpha-linolenic acid). Both DHA and ALA are omega-3 fatty acids, but DHA is particularly important for neurological function—there is more DHA in your brain than any other fatty acid. So if you take curcumin with your omega-3s, more of the ALA may be converted to DHA.
- Using turmeric in recipes can help some foods better retain their beta-carotene during the cooking process.
- Many produce sections now offer raw turmeric root, often kept near the gingerroot. In fact, turmeric root resembles gingerroot but is more yellow-orange in color. I recommend buying nonirradiated herbs and spices, and whenever possible, buy organic.
- Dried turmeric powder should be kept in a tightly sealed container in a cool, dark, and dry place. Fresh turmeric root should be stored in the refrigerator.
- Turmeric powder can also be taken in supplement form, especially if you need to achieve therapeutic levels. I personally recommend a carbon dioxide–extracted form of turmeric.
- If you combine your turmeric with a little black pepper, the turmeric may be more usable throughout your body, thanks to a compound in

black pepper called piperine. In one study, adding 20 milligrams of piperine to 2,000 milligrams of turmeric increased its bioavailability by 154 percent.
* One study found that when curcumin is combined with the steroid medication prednisolone, the side effects of the medication were significantly reduced.

Be a Fat Flush Cook
* Turmeric can make your grilled meat safer by helping prevent formation of heterocyclic amines. A teaspoon or two of turmeric per 3½ ounces of meat was used to produce this helpful outcome in one study, as well as satay marinated in a turmeric-containing spice mixture.
* My favorite way to enjoy turmeric is in a hot turmeric toddy at bedtime, which helps me relax. Simply combine one cup of almond milk with a quarter of a teaspoon of ginger, an eighth of a teaspoon of Ceylon cinnamon, and half a teaspoon of ground turmeric. Bring the brew to a boil, simmer three minutes, and relax knowing all those power nutrients are doing wonderful things in your body as you sleep.

Fat Flush Fun
* Besides culinary and medicinal applications, turmeric has been used throughout history as a fabric dye.
* You can add turmeric powder to playdough to make marigold-colored playdough, and it works as a natural Easter egg dye too.
* Many swear by turmeric as a dandruff and scalp tonic! Just mix turmeric with the oil of your choice (olive, jojoba, and/or coconut oil work well), massage into your scalp, and leave in for 15 minutes. Then just shampoo and style as usual. As warned above, turmeric can stain towels, so proceed with caution!

THINK TWICE!
* *There have been a few allergic reactions documented from turmeric. According to reports, some people have developed a mild, itchy rash from skin exposure. Other reports include instances of nausea, diarrhea, hypotension, increased bleeding risk, hyperactive gallbladder contractions, increased menstrual flow, and uterine contractions in pregnant women.*
* *The intense pigments in turmeric will stain almost anything—sometimes permanently! So watch out with your clothes, towels, countertops, and kitchen wares.*

6 Surprising Fat Flush Foods

To eat is a necessity, but to eat intelligently is an art.

—La Rochefoucauld

In this chapter, you'll find foods that have earned a place on your Fat Flush dinner plate. Some of my selections may surprise you, because they are items often omitted from the typical dieter's grocery list. However, each of these foods provides concentrated nutrition—giving you the best Fat Flush bang for your buck.

For example, I recommend whole-fat yogurt, rather than the fat-free varieties that are so often loaded with extra carbs and artificial sweeteners. Along with those all-important active bacterial cultures, yogurt provides calcium, which is emerging as one of the latest weight loss tools. You will also find shirataki noodles, yacon syrup, and tigernut flour—those exotic-sounding but delicious and versatile foods to add to your shopping list. All of these assist in weight control and satiety by providing high fiber and probiotic power.

You have the power to reach your weight loss goals by eating the right kinds of fat-flushing fats, proteins, and carbohydrates. The key to achieving a fit, toned body is to start from the inside out by cleansing the liver, revving up the metabolism, and evening out blood sugar levels. Only then will your body be primed for optimal fat burning and weight loss. The following eight foods make important contributions to your development as a lean, mean fat-burning machine.

ALMONDS

> ### Fat Flush Factors
>
> *Blood Sugar Stabilizer*
> *Cholesterol Zapper*
> *Energizer*

What blooms like a peach and looks like a peach, but is harvested for its seed rather than its fruit? You guessed it—it's the almond. These oval, off-white nuts grow on trees and are technically the seeds of almond fruits. One of the earliest cultivated foods, the almond is the most nutritionally well-balanced nut. It is high in protein, contains healthy fats, and offers ample amounts of vitamin E, calcium, fiber, folate, iron, potassium, zinc, and magnesium. But there's more. Almonds are an excellent source of biotin, a B vitamin involved in the metabolism of both sugar and fat. By eating almonds, you can boost your energy, improve the health of your skin and hair, and maximize your nervous system function.

Studies have shown that people who eat almonds on a regular basis enjoy a lower risk of heart disease, have healthy blood sugar levels, and have a good chance of shedding those excess pounds. A recent study, published by the American Heart Association, detailed the effect that almonds can have on cholesterol levels. Dieters who ate two handfuls of almonds per day saw a drop in LDL cholesterol levels of over 9 percent, compared with dieters who substituted a low-fat, whole wheat muffin for the almonds. Many researchers agree that crunching on an ounce of almonds per day will reduce your risk of heart disease by 30 percent.

Because almonds contain fiber, protein, and fat, they satisfy both your appetite and the desire for something crunchy. Snacking on a small handful of almonds can help you feel fuller, longer. A recent study followed 65 overweight people, three-fourths of whom were type 2 diabetics. The group of dieters who ate 3 ounces of almonds every day dropped 18 percent of their weight in 24 weeks. The dieters who ate the same healthy menu, without the almonds, averaged only an 11 percent loss. In addition to the faster weight loss, the almond eaters saw improvement in their blood pressure readings and were able to lower their use of diabetes medications. It's unmistakable. Almonds are a high-fat food that is great for your health and your waistline.

Recommended Usage

Up to one ounce of almonds per day.

Just the Facts

- How long have almonds been around? Botanists believe they are a *prehistoric* hybrid of unknown origins.
- California produces 80 percent of the world's supply of almonds.
- If you cut down an almond tree, shoots grow up from the stump and become a tree again in just a few years.
- One-fourth cup of almonds contains more protein than an egg.

Boost the Benefits

- Since almonds have a high fat content, they must be stored properly to protect them from becoming rancid. *Unshelled* almonds have the longest shelf life. When buying these, avoid shells that are split, moldy, or stained.
- Because they are not exposed to heat, air, and humidity, shelled almonds that come in a sealed container will last longer than those sold in bulk bins. When you're buying almonds from bulk bins, look for nuts with a uniform color. Avoid almonds that are limp or shriveled or have a sharp or bitter odor. Store almonds in sealed plastic bags or glass jars. If well sealed, you can refrigerate almonds for several months, or you can pop them in the freezer for up to one year.
- If you combine almonds with foods rich in vitamin C, you'll improve your body's ability to absorb iron.
- Give your bones a boost. Eating approximately 20 almonds provides you with as much calcium as one-quarter cup of milk.

Just for Fun!

- A favorite snack among Japanese teenagers is a mixture of dried sardines and slivered almonds.

Be a Fat Flush Cook

- To toast your own almonds, spread them in a shallow pan and heat them in a 170 degree oven for 20 minutes. This preserves the healthy oils in the nuts.
- Sprinkle some chopped almonds over a salad or steamed vegetables.
- Skip that high-carb granola and mix some chopped almonds into your yogurt instead.

- Add crunch to your stir-fry with a handful of sliced almonds.
- A spoonful of natural almond butter added to your morning smoothie gives it extra flavor and protein.

THINK TWICE!

- Nuts can cause hives, headaches, and other allergic reactions. People who are allergic to aspirin may react to the natural salicylates found in almonds.
- The commercial roasting process for nuts is a form of deep frying, usually in saturated fat such as coconut or palm kernel oil. If you buy roasted almonds, select ones that have been "dry roasted." Check the label to be sure that no additional ingredients such as sugar, corn syrup, or preservatives have been added.

IT'S BEEN SAID . . .

I'm always looking for a healthy snack that I can pack in my purse. My latest favorite is slivered almonds and apple slices.

SUSAN T., IOWA

OLIVE OIL

Fat Flush Factors

Blood Sugar Stabilizer
Cholesterol Zapper
Detoxifier

Since ancient times, the olive tree has served as a symbol of peace and has supplied people with food, fuel, and medicine. While olive oil has been consumed since 3000 BC, it enjoyed little popularity in the United States until the 1970s. During that decade, researchers began to boast about the health benefits of olive oil, causing supermarkets to carry a sampling of olive oils from various countries.

Today, on grocery shelves, you can find a number of grades of olive oil—ranging from "premium extra virgin" to "light." Premium extra virgin olive oil is produced by pressing perfectly ripe olives within 24 hours of their being harvested. It contains the highest density of powerful antioxidants called polyphenols, known for attacking free radicals before they can do their cholesterol-raising damage.

Extra virgin olive oil is made from the first pressing of olives, while virgin olive oil comes from olives that are slightly riper. Pure olive oil is a commercial-grade blend of olive pulp, skins, and pits. Light olive oil results from the final pressing of a batch of olives and carries little of the true aroma and flavor of olive oil.

Although olive oil is a fat, it still ranks as a Fat Flush food. It deserves this status because of its monounsaturated fat, which decreases LDL cholesterol and the risk of heart disease. In addition, the natural antioxidants in olive oil help lower cholesterol levels, maintain a healthy blood pressure, and guard against the toxins that can cause breast cancer.

Because of its low acidity level, especially in the higher grades of oil, olive oil is easier to digest compared with most other fats. The high vitamin E content of olives may even help reduce the frequency and intensity of hot flashes in women going through menopause. And by consuming small amounts of this good fat, you'll help satisfy your appetite and keep your blood sugar on an even keel.

Recommended Usage

Up to one tablespoon per day.

Just the Facts

- In ancient Greece, olive oil was so highly valued that only virgin boys were allowed to pick olives, one by one.
- Spain is the world's biggest supplier of olive oil. Some of its olive trees are over 1,000 years old.
- Olive oil is always of the best quality in the year it is produced, unlike wine, which may require several years to reach its peak.
- The cost of extra virgin olive oil ranges from $5 to $100 per quart, depending on the type of olive used, where it was cultivated, and how it was processed.

Boost the Benefits

- Air, heat, and light cause olive oil to turn rancid, so store it in a cool, dark place in a container with a tight cap. If you refrigerate it, the oil may thicken and darken, but it will return to its original, liquid state when it is warmed to room temperature. However, refrigeration may alter the flavor of extra virgin oil, so treat it delicately.
- Once you've opened a bottle of olive oil, it begins to oxidize and is best when used within a couple of months. However, if it is stored properly, olive oil can be kept longer than any other edible oil without going rancid.
- Your best bet is to store olive oil in a glass, glazed clay, or stainless-steel container. Copper or iron containers cause a chemical reaction, which damages the oil and may produce toxins. Avoid storing olive oil in plastic containers because, over time, the oil can absorb some of the compounds used in the plastic.
- Because of the higher acidity level, lower grades of olive oil have a shorter shelf life than top-quality extra virgin oil.

Be a Fat Flush Cook

- Olive oil is perfect for meat, fish, or poultry marinades. Brushing olive oil onto meats prior to broiling, grilling, or roasting will help brown the meat and seal in the juices.
- Instead of serving butter with bread, pour a bit of olive oil onto a small plate for dipping.
- Sprinkle olive oil on cooked vegetables for a satisfying flavor.

- Substituting light olive oil for butter makes for moist and tender baked goods, without risk of a heavy olive flavor. For most recipes, use three-fourths of a cup oil for every cup of butter.
- Tossing vegetables in olive oil before cooking seals in moisture, adds flavor, and promotes browning.
- For sautéing or baking, use light olive oil, but when mixing a salad dressing, extra virgin olive oil is worth every penny.

THINK TWICE!

- *Some flavored olive oils have additives that require refrigeration in order to preserve them, so please read the label carefully. If you make your own flavored olive oils, use them immediately, because some flavoring agents promote the growth of bacteria.*
- *If you purchase unfiltered olive oil, it should be consumed within a year of production. Keep in mind that it takes some time for olive oil to reach store shelves, so six months may have passed by the time you buy it.*
- *Some people experience a slight laxative effect from olive oil, so add it gradually to your daily diet.*

Fat Flush Fun

- If you want to taste-test olive oil like the experts, follow these simple steps:
  - Pour one tablespoon of olive oil in a small glass. Rotate the glass delicately until the oil has adhered to the entire inside surface of the glass. Warm the glass in your hands until it is close to body temperature.
  - Lift the glass to your nose and sniff rapidly and deeply three times. Try to analyze the aroma.
  - Take a small sip but don't swallow! Roll the olive oil around in your mouth for a few seconds; then spit it out. A low-quality oil will leave an aftertaste, while high-quality extra virgin olive oil will leave your mouth clean, with just a hint of pepper.
  - If you are sampling more than one oil, drink lots of water and eat a small piece of bread between samples.

IT'S BEEN SAID . . .

While on a Fat Flush Caribbean Cruise with Ann Louise, she told us how great olive oil is for the skin. She rubs olive oil on her elbows and into her cuticles. Give it a try—it really works!

LINDA L., DURHAM, NC

QUINOA

Fat Flush Factors
Blood Sugar Stabilizer
Cholesterol Zapper
Detoxifier
Energizer

Quinoa (pronounced "keen-wah") has become a favorite of many wanting to avoid the pitfalls of grain. Its botanical name is *Chenopodium quinoa*, which is not a grain but rather a seed—a tiny nutritional powerhouse with tons of fiber, protein, and antioxidants. Quinoa has been shown to benefit blood sugar and lipid levels. This little seed is fabulous for anyone on a gluten-free diet because so few are allergic to it—it doesn't even come from the same family as wheat, oats, barley, or rye.

This interesting plant was first cultivated by the Incas more than 5,000 years ago and remains largely unchanged today. High up in the Andes, quinoa plants have overcome the challenges of high altitude, intense heat, freezing temperatures, and sparse rainfall. The plants resemble spinach but sport towering magenta stalks with huge flashy seed heads in a rainbow of colors—red, purple, pink, and yellow. There are literally hundreds of quinoa cultivars.

If you're a vegetarian, quinoa is invaluable because it's a complete protein, having all nine essential amino acids. It also contains a high percentage of protein—to a tune of six grams per quarter cup, which is more than wheat, rice, or millet. This ancient food also contains twice the fiber of most grains.

When it comes to fats, quinoa has more than most grains with about 25 percent being in the form of oleic acid, a monounsaturated fat offering cardiovascular benefits. Quinoa also has some alpha-linolenic acid, the omega-3 fat most often provided by plants. Despite these fats, the process of boiling, simmering, or steaming quinoa does not appear to compromise the quality of its fatty acids. Quinoa is also rich in manganese, magnesium, copper, phosphorous, folate, zinc, riboflavin (vitamin B2), and oodles of antioxidants—outperforming grains by a country mile.

Brazilian scientists recently researched 10 traditional Peruvian "grains" and legumes for their potential in managing the early stages of type 2 diabetes. They discovered quinoa is especially rich in an antioxidant called quercetin and had the highest overall antioxidant activity of all 10 foods examined. Quercetin inhibits histamine release, making quercetin-rich foods natural antihistamines.

Quinoa was also found to contain kaempferol, which combats cancer and lowers your heart disease risk. Quinoa's concentration of quercetin and kaempferol is even higher than in high-flavonoid berries like cranberry and lingonberry—which really says something! Quinoa also contains substantial phenolic acids (for anti-inflammatory benefits) and other phytonutrients including ferulic, coumaric, hydroxybenzoic, and vanillic acids.

This seed's nutritional bounty will significantly benefit your heart and help protect you from type 2 diabetes. In one study, those consuming quinoa reduced their triglyceride levels more than those consuming other gluten-free products. Another study showed that quinoa may help mitigate the damage from eating a high-fructose diet in terms of lipid and glucose levels.

Although preliminary, recent studies all point to quinoa's enormous anti-inflammatory benefits, including gut inflammation. The saponins on the exterior of quinoa seeds exert both anti-inflammatory and antioxidant effects. The plant produces this bitter coating to repel and kill insects. Quinoa is a friendly carbohydrate you can use in any recipe that calls for rice. Even Fat Flush–friendly quinoa noodles have recently popped up on market shelves!

Recommended Usage

- Just like a grain, quinoa can be milled and ground into a flour for use in cookies, muffins, breads, and other gluten-free baking fun. It can even be popped like popcorn, a treat enjoyed by Peruvian children.
- Sprouted quinoa can be used in soups, salads, and sandwiches, just like alfalfa and other sprouts.
- Quinoa can be used in place of rice in any recipe. Now that quinoa noodles are available, you can have pasta again!
- Try mixing cooked quinoa into your hamburger, meatball, or meatloaf mix in place of bread crumbs.
- Quinoa works well hot, cold, or halfway in between. It can even be used as a breakfast grain. Mixing cinnamon, nuts, and/or fruit into cooked quinoa turns it into a hearty breakfast porridge.
- Quinoa makes a marvelous wheat-free alternative in the Middle Eastern dish tabouli, which traditionally calls for bulgur wheat. Or try this: toss cooked quinoa with black beans, pumpkin seeds, scallions, and coriander for a lovely dish packed with protein, fiber, and antioxidants that will keep you going for hours.

Just the Facts

- For thousands of years, quinoa has been a dietary staple in South America. It was first cultivated by the Inca in the high Andes as far back as 5,000 years ago. The sweetest-tasting quinoa is that grown above 12,500 feet.
- Not realizing its value, Spanish conquistadors nearly wiped out quinoa in the New World by making it illegal for native Indians to grow. Fortunately, a small amount survived and in the 1980s, two Americans rediscovered the crop and began growing it in Colorado. Now, more than 200,000 pounds are grown in the Rocky Mountains every year. However, most of the quinoa consumed in the United States still comes from South America, with Peru being its largest producer.

Boost the Benefits

- The saponins on quinoa can impart a slightly bitter flavor. However, saponins are easily removed by rinsing the quinoa in water before cooking. Although most packaged quinoas have already undergone a rinsing, it's never a bad idea to give them an extra rinse. Simply place the quinoa in a strainer and run cold water over it until the soapy residue (saponin) is washed away.
- Saponins were used by native South American peoples to promote skin healing and were thought to be a good antiseptic.
- Quinoa is best stored in an airtight container in the refrigerator where it will keep for three to six months.

Be a Fat Flush Cook

- To prepare quinoa, add one part quinoa seeds to two parts liquid (water or bone broth) in a saucepan. Bring to a boil and then lower the heat to "simmer" and cover the pan. One cup of quinoa typically takes just 15 minutes to cook. You will know it's done when the grains become translucent and the white germ has partially detached itself, looking almost like a tiny white curly tail.
- Cooked quinoa seeds are fluffy and creamy, yet also slightly crunchy, and have a delicate nutty flavor. To bring out more nuttiness, you can dry-roast your quinoa before cooking it. Simply place the seeds in a dry skillet over medium-low heat and stir constantly for five minutes; then cook as usual.

THINK TWICE!

- *Quinoa is not a commonly allergenic food, but it does contain oxalates, so consume it with caution if you are on an oxalate-restricted diet.*
- *Saponins have been known to cause a little stomach irritation among those particularly susceptible.*

Fat Flush Fun

- Saponins prevent birds from eating quinoa seeds off the bushes. Scientists decided to create a quinoa without saponins, and guess what happened: the birds ate it all!
- Many South Americans use quinoa-derived saponin as a detergent for washing their clothes. They also use pigments (betacyanin) from the colorful leaves of the plant to dye their textiles, producing some lovely flashy red hues.

IT'S BEEN SAID . . .

The Inca referred to quinoa as the "mother seed" and considered it sacred.

SHIRATAKI NOODLES

Fat Flush Factors

Blood Sugar Stabilizer
Cholesterol Zapper

If you've been testing out low-carb diets over the past several years, you've probably run across shirataki noodles—or "miracle noodles" as one company has dubbed them. Any pasta lover trying to curb carbohydrate cravings would agree that a nutritious zero-calorie noodle totally rocks the concept of miraculous!

Shirataki noodles are made from glucomannan fiber, which is derived from the root of the konjac plant (*Amorphophallus konjac*), also known as devil's tongue yam. These long, whitish-translucent noodles are widely used in China and Japan and contain 97 percent water, 3 percent fiber, and close to zero calories with no digestible carbs. Glucomannan fiber is a biochemical mix of the two sugars mannose and glucose. Shirataki noodles also offer at least 16 amino acids and a montage of minerals and vitamins.

One great benefit of these noodles is that they are highly satisfying, despite contributing almost no calories or carbohydrates to your meal. What explains this magic? Resistant starch. Fiber is typically classified as either soluble or insoluble, but when it comes to health benefits, there are other important distinctions, such as fermentability. Glucomannan is a type of resistant starch—in other words, a starch that resists digestion in your small intestine. This type of fiber makes it into your lower digestive tract where it is fermented by your gut flora, meaning it's a natural prebiotic. Keeping your microbiome happy and healthy allows it to perform important anti-inflammatory, immune, and metabolic processes.

When the microorganisms in your gut ferment resistant starch, beneficial by-products are created, including short-chain fatty acids (butyrate, propionate, acetate) that calibrate your immune system and serve as a substrate for ketone production and fuel for your mitochondria—which translates into increased energy for you!

One unique property of glucomannan fiber is that it swells to about 17 times its original volume when combined with water. In your digestive tract, it forms a gelatinous mass that slows down digestion and keeps you feeling fuller longer. Because resistant starches are fermented very slowly, they (usually) won't make you gassy. As you might expect, shirataki noodles bulk up the stool and help you maintain regular bowel movements.

Glucomannan has been found to increase satiety hormones and reduce levels of ghrelin, the "hunger hormone." Resistant starch has been proved to assist weight loss, stabilize blood sugar, reduce inflammation, lower LDL, and produce other healthy metabolic effects. Research also suggests that resistant starch may help prevent leaky gut, lower your risk for colon cancer, reduce serum thyroid levels in those with hyperthyroidism, and possibly even slow the effects of aging.

If you haven't yet tried shirataki noodles, you owe it to yourself to do so! They are virtually tasteless themselves, but they take on the flavors of the foods they're combined with, a bit like tofu. Not only are shirataki noodles a godsend for Fat Flushers, but they're a valuable addition for anyone on gluten-free, reduced-carb, and other dietary protocols.

Recommended Usage

- Because shirataki noodles readily take on the flavor of whatever seasoning or sauce you put them with, they are lovely in broth, especially flavorful homemade bone broth. Ramen will never be the same again! They also don't stick together like standard grain-based noodles.
- Shirataki require very little in the way of preparation—you don't even have to cook them. Simply rinse, drain, and dress with your favorite seasoning or sauce. Rinsing them removes the slightly fishy smell associated with konjac.
- Shirataki have a crunchy-like texture. If you prefer a more "noodly" texture, heat them in an ungreased skillet for a few minutes.
- Shirataki are also available as a rice.
- Glucomannan starch is sold as a powder that can be used to thicken sauces, gravies, puddings, etc., without affecting taste. Just be careful—it's 10 times as potent for thickening as cornstarch! Use too much, and you'll get something like wallpaper paste.

Just the Facts

- The word *shirataki* means "white waterfall," as the noodles are thin, translucent, and gelatinous. Traditional Chinese and Japanese cuisine has incorporated konjac for over 2,000 years.
- The konjac plant grows mainly in southwest China mountain ranges— the region where pandas live! The root of the plant is full of fiber, which is the part used to make konjac foods.
- Glucomannan has the highest molecular weight of any dietary fiber known to science. When you pick up a bag of shirataki noodles, you'll notice how heavy they are.

- Glucomannan also has the highest water-holding capacity of any soluble fiber—it can hold 100 times its own weight in water.
- The noodles are sold in airtight bags that can be stored at room temperature (in your pantry) for about a year. They don't require refrigeration.

Boost the Benefits

- Are you nutsy for noodles? Besides shirataki, there are other nice low-carb pasta alternatives. Kelp noodles are similar to shirataki but made from brown seaweed, instead of konjac. They contain only kelp, sodium alginate (a seaweed-derived salt), and water, and they're rich in minerals and iodine. Kelp noodles are even crunchier than shirataki—almost having a "squeaky" mouth feel. However, some say dousing them in something acidic tames them down a bit, such as lime juice or tomato sauce.
- Ancient Harvest makes some fabulous high-protein red lentil, supergrain, and quinoa pastas.
- Don't forget about vegetable noodles such as spaghetti squash and spiralized zucchini.

THINK TWICE!

- *In some people, glucomannan can trigger a few intestinal symptoms such as loose stools, diarrhea, or flatulence. Those who experience this can usually find relief just by reducing the quantity a bit.*

SWEET POTATOES

> ## Fat Flush Factors
>
> **Blood Sugar Stabilizer**
> **Cholesterol Zapper**

It's hard to believe that a food with both "sweet" and "potato" in its name is a great food for dieters. Yet it's true. Sweet potatoes are among the most nutritious foods in the vegetable kingdom. And as scientists have discovered, they are also one of the oldest-known vegetables, having been consumed 10,000 years ago by prehistoric people.

In the early 1900s, Americans were most familiar with the pale-fleshed sweet potato. When a new orange-colored variety was introduced, it was frequently called a "yam" to avoid confusion between the two types of sweet potatoes. However, a true yam is a large African root vegetable that can grow to be 100 pounds and is rarely found in the United States.

Despite its name, the sweet potato bears no relation to the common potato and can be eaten by people who normally steer clear of potatoes. Sweet potatoes are packed with calcium, potassium, and vitamins A, C, and E. They also provide fiber, iron, thiamine, and manganese. As an antioxidant-rich food, the sweet potato helps the body eliminate free radicals, chemicals that damage cells and promote heart disease and cancer.

Recently, sweet potatoes gained the well-deserved title of "antidiabetic food" because of their power to stabilize blood sugar levels and lower insulin resistance. So the next time your sweet tooth rears its ugly head, skip the cakes and cookies and enjoy a delicious and satisfying sweet potato.

Recommended Usage

Two to three ½-cup servings per week.

Just the Facts

- Sweet potatoes contain an enzyme that contributes to its sugary flavor. This sweetness continues to increase during storage and as the potatoes are cooked.
- Despite their sweetness, sweet potatoes are considerably lower on the glycemic index than white potatoes. A baked sweet potato is 77 on the index, while a baked white potato is 121.

- Out of 400 varieties of sweet potatoes, 2 are most common: the pale-yellow kind with dry flesh and those that are dark orange with a moist flesh. Generally, dark-orange sweet potatoes are plumper and more flavorful.
- During the Civil War, coffee was scarce, so people dried sweet potatoes and ground them as a substitute for coffee.
- While sweet potatoes can be found year-round, they are in season during November and December.

Boost the Benefits

- When you're buying sweet potatoes, select potatoes that are heavy and firm with smooth, bright skin and no cracks or bruises. Avoid potatoes on display in a refrigerated produce section because the cold can be damaging.
- Keep in mind that even if you cut away a spot of decay, it may have already given the whole potato an unpleasant flavor.
- Store sweet potatoes in a cool, dark, and well-ventilated place. Temperatures above 60 degrees cause them to sprout or ferment, while air cooler than 50 degrees triggers an unpleasant change in flavor. Keep the potatoes loose, not in a plastic bag, and they should remain fresh for at least 10 days.
- Before storing sweet potatoes, you may brush off excess dirt, but to prevent spoilage, do not wash them until you are ready to cook them.
- Cook sweet potatoes *whole* whenever possible since most of the nutrients are next to the skin. However, because dyes and wax are sometimes used on the skin, do not eat it unless the potato has been grown organically.

Be a Fat Flush Cook

- Yellow and orange sweet potatoes may be used interchangeably in recipes; however, avoid mixing the two types, as their cooking times vary.
- Puree cooked sweet potatoes with a bit of natural applesauce and cinnamon. Top with ground flax seed.
- Cut a sweet potato into thin slices and bake to make crunchy sweet potato chips.
- Sweet potatoes can be boiled, grilled, baked, or roasted. So don't be afraid to experiment with this versatile vegetable.
- You can freeze cooked sweet potatoes. Simply add a little lemon juice to prevent darkening and pack them into freezer containers.

THINK TWICE!

- *While canned sweet potatoes are available, they usually come in heavy syrup and are substantially lower in beta-carotene, vitamin C, and B vitamins than fresh ones.*
- *Because pesticide residues are commonly found on sweet potatoes, it's best to look for organically grown ones whenever possible.*
- *Sweet potatoes are among the few foods that contain oxalates, which, if concentrated in the body, can crystallize and cause health problems. If you have a history of kidney or gallbladder trouble, you may want to avoid eating sweet potatoes.*
- *Oxalates may also prevent the body from absorbing calcium. If you take calcium supplements, allow two to three hours between taking your supplement and eating a sweet potato.*

IT'S BEEN SAID . . .

I'm always looking for new things to pack for lunch. My latest favorite is a sweet potato, baked the night before and packed cold in my lunch bag. Yum! It's almost like having dessert.

JENNIFER B., FLORIDA

TIGERNUTS

> ### Fat Flush Factors
> *Blood Sugar Stabilizer*
> *Cholesterol Zapper*
> *Energizer*

One of the greatest foods to hit the markets recently is tigernuts. It's hard to imagine a friendlier carbohydrate—not to mention a more versatile one! Ground tigernuts make for a handy high-fiber flour substitute, and tigernut oil is delicious drizzled on salads, cooked veggies, or meats. Tigernuts can even be used to make a tasty traditional beverage called horchata, a nondairy milk substitute that gives coconut, almond, and soy milk a run for their money.

Tigernuts can be snacked on like a nut . . . but they are not actually a nut, so they're perfect for those with nut allergies. Tigernuts (*Cyperus esculentus*) are the tuberous root of a wild grass originating on the African continent. You can't get any more "Paleo" than that, as recent researchers suggest tigernuts may have been the original "trail mix." Early hominids consumed large quantities of these little bulbs found at the base of grass blades. They grow much like a potato, in underground clusters knit together by fine root filaments.

The nutritional profile of tigernuts is a combination of beneficial starches, fiber, monounsaturated fats, amino acids, vitamins, minerals, and enzymes. Tigernuts are about 33 percent fiber, and gram for gram, they contain almost six times as much sugar as sweet potatoes, yet amazingly still boast a low glycemic index value.

Tigernuts are packed with resistant starch that is digested slowly, acting as a prebiotic that nourishes the good bacteria of your digestive tract. Prebiotics help your body flush out harmful, inflammation-producing organisms and replace them with the beneficial ones that stabilize blood glucose levels, increase insulin sensitivity, and help prevent obesity. Resistant starch also increases butyrate production in your gut. Butyrate is the preferred energy source for the cells lining your colon and plays supportive roles in metabolism, inflammation, and stress mitigation.

Tigernut fat is 73 percent monounsaturated in the form of oleic acid (anti-inflammatory, supporting good HDL), 18 percent saturated fat (also anti-inflammatory), but only 9 percent polyunsaturated fat as linoleic acid (pro-inflammatory). Tigernuts are also packed with magnesium and argi-nine, an amino acid that optimizes your blood flow by increasing nitric oxide production and hence vasodilation. So these little tubers are awe-somely heart healthy!

In addition to magnesium, tigernuts provide a wealth of calcium, potassium, iron, phosphorous, zinc, copper, and vitamins C and E, as well as glutamic acid (important for neurotransmitters and brain health), aspartic acid (cellular energy and metabolism), and digestive enzymes including catalase, lipase, and amylase. As for flavor, tigernuts are pleas-antly sweet with an almost caramel flavor that's milder than that of most nuts. In today's fast-paced world, it's nice to have snacks we can grab in a hurry that won't send our blood sugar soaring—and tigernuts fit the bill. As Tony the Tiger would say, "They're grrrrreat!"

Recommended Usage
- Tigernuts can be consumed raw or roasted.
- Tigernut flour makes a suitable one-to-one replacement for wheat flour in most recipes.
- Chewing tigernuts whole is a bit like chewing up the stem of a partic-ularly fibrous stalk of asparagus, a texture some may find objection-able. However, their flavor is absolutely divine!

Just the Facts
- Tigernuts are one of the oldest cultivated plants in ancient Egypt. They grow primarily in tropical and Mediterranean regions and are a traditional food in Nigeria.
- Tigernut plants are also called chufa (in Spain), nut grass, yellow nutsedge, chufa sedge, or earth almond.
- Tigernuts have been used medicinally for millennia including orally and topically and have even been used as enemas. Dry tubers have been found in tombs dating back 6,000 years.
- Tigernuts may act as an aphrodisiac.
- Feel free to slather your skin in tigernut oil. Because it's so rich in vita-min E, tigernut oil is now being used by the cosmetic industry.

Boost the Benefits
- Tigernuts can be stored at room temperature.

Be a Fat Flush Cook

• Popular in Spain, a drink called horchata de chufa (or in Nigeria, kunnu aya) is becoming popular out West. You can make your own horchata by blending the milky extract of tigernuts with water (plus optional spices and sweeteners). It's essentially the same process as for making nut milks.

• The website Nourished Kitchen offers a simple horchata recipe, which produces about one quart:
   – *Ingredients:* Eight ounces of raw organic tigernuts, one quart of filtered water, one cinnamon stick, three cardamom pods, and the sweetener of your choice (stevia, Lakanto, dates, etc.). Keep in mind that tigernuts are naturally sweet—much more so than almond or coconut milk—so you may not need any sweetener.
   – *Instructions:* Soak the tigernuts and cinnamon stick in water for 12 to 24 hours to soften. Using a high-power blender, blend the mixture into a smooth paste, adding water as necessary to facilitate the blending. Spoon the mixture into a nut milk bag and press through. Add enough water to produce a drinkable consistency.

THINK TWICE!

• *As with any new food, start with just a few tigernuts and see how you feel. Occasionally, resistant starches can cause a little gas, bloating, or diarrhea, which is usually dose related.*

YACON SYRUP

Fat Flush Factors

Blood Sugar Stabilizer
Energizer

Yacon syrup, also called yacon nectar, is a natural low-glycemic sweetener made from a tuber that's naturally high in prebiotics, including inulin and fructooligosaccharides (FOS). Unlike most roots, which are quite starchy, yacon stores its sugars as FOS rather than starch, accounting for its sweeter taste. In fact, yacon is thought to be the richest source of FOS in the natural world.

If you're not familiar with the benefits of FOS, then here's a short primer. Fructooligosaccharides resist breakdown by your digestive enzymes, so they reach your colon intact. Yacon's FOS and inulin are sources of soluble fiber that feed the beneficial bacteria in your gut, helping them perform their important anti-inflammatory, immune, and metabolic roles. They convert FOS into short-chain fatty acids that benefit your lipid profile and insulin response, among other things. The FOS and inulin in yacon also bulk up your stool, making FOS an effective remedy for constipation.

Additionally, FOS modulates gastric emptying, increasing satiety and decreasing food cravings, and this is especially beneficial for those battling metabolic syndrome or type 2 diabetes. Yacon has also been shown to decrease fat accumulation in the liver, as well as having anti-cancer potential.

A 2009 study of yacon syrup for weight loss sparked a great deal of excitement and controversy. Researchers conducted a double-blind, placebo-controlled study involving 55 women. Those consuming yacon syrup as part of a restricted-calorie, low-fat diet experienced dramatic weight loss—averaging 33 pounds in four months—whereas the placebo group actually gained 3 pounds. The yacon group also lost inches and improved their BMI, insulin levels, and LDL. Further studies will need to be done, but this was certainly encouraging.

Yacon is rich in calcium, potassium, and phosphorous and has been shown to boost mineral absorption. The calcium in yacon is highly bioavailable, supporting healthy bones. Studies show that yacon and other fructans may also offer immune benefits such as staving off infections and reducing allergies.

Yacon syrup is similar in color and consistency to molasses, but milder in flavor. The leaves of the plant can be brewed into an antioxidant-rich tea, but the root can also be eaten raw like jicama or roasted like potatoes.

The syrup is about three-quarters as sweet as honey, but because a large portion moves through your GI tract undigested, it has only one-third of the calories of honey—20 calories per tablespoon compared with 64 for honey. Although yacon syrup is almost half FOS, it does contain some sugars, and so it's best consumed in moderation. The nutritional breakdown of the syrup (raw) is as follows: FOS 47 percent, water 22 percent, sucrose 20 percent, fructose 7 percent, glucose 3 percent, and protein 1 percent. Yacon syrup is allowed on phase 3 of my New Fat Flush Plan.

Recommended Usage

- Yacon syrup is delightful in tea and salad dressings. Its flavor profile mingles particularly well with apple cider vinegar.
- Raw yacon root has a pleasantly crunchy, juicy texture, a bit like water chestnuts.
- The root can be peeled, grated, or sliced and then added to salads. It's also delicious as a raw snack, sliced into sticks like jicama.
- Yacon root can be added to stir-fries, steamed, or even roasted with other root vegetables.

Just the Facts

- Yacon syrup comes from the plant *Smallanthus sonchifolius* (previously *Polymnia sonchifolial*), native to the Andes Mountains of South America. It's a member of the Asteraceae family, a cousin to sunflowers, dahlias, Jerusalem artichokes, and other common plants.
- Cultivation may date back as far as 1200 BC.
- Due to the rising popularity of yacon syrup, yacon is now grown in many regions across the globe—even home gardeners are growing it. Yacon will grow anywhere Jerusalem artichokes grow.

Boost the Benefits

- When yacon syrup is thermally processed, much of the FOS converts to sugar, and so you lose a large part of its nutritional value. For this reason, make sure you purchase pure, raw organic yacon syrup that's free of additives. To qualify as "raw," the processing temperatures must not exceed about 104 degrees Fahrenheit.

• Experts suggest that consuming yacon syrup 30 to 60 minutes before a meal may tamp down appetite.

Fat Flush in Action

• If you are planning to use raw yacon root in salad or as a snack, dipping the peeled and sliced roots in water acidified with lemon juice or apple cider vinegar helps prevent discoloration.

THINK TWICE!

• *In some individuals, yacon can cause flatulence, nausea, diarrhea, or other digestive discomforts. If you have a sensitive digestive system or tend toward loose stools, then you might want to avoid yacon or at least proceed with caution to see how you react.*

Fat Flush Fun

• *Yacon* means "water root" in the Inca language.
• In historical times, yacon tubers were valued as a source of thirst-quenching refreshment for parched and weary travelers.
• If you have a garden, try growing your own yacon as detailed on the University of California Master Gardener's website. Then take the next step by making your own syrup!

YOGURT

Fat Flush Factors
Detoxifier
Energizer
Thermogenic

Yogurt is one dairy product that I can recommend wholeheartedly. Made by adding bacterial cultures to milk, yogurt has a refreshingly tart flavor and a unique creamy texture. Because it contains beneficial bacteria, yogurt increases resistance to immune-related diseases and may help you live longer. One recent five-year study tracked a population of 162 very elderly people and found that those who ate yogurt more than three times per week were 38 percent more likely to survive the term of the study than those who ate yogurt less than once a week.

Yogurt provides ample amounts of a number of important nutrients. If you consume yogurt regularly, you'll be strengthening your bones with calcium and phosphorous, fortifying body tissues with protein, and energizing your metabolism with riboflavin and niacin. But it is the bacterial cultures—known as probiotics—that make yogurt a Fat Flush superfood.

From minimizing bad breath to preventing yeast infections, probiotics work their magic throughout the body. They contribute to intestinal health, and because they are resistant to stomach acid, they continue their beneficial activities as they travel through the entire digestive tract. Johns Hopkins researchers found that yogurt helps reduce fatty liver disease, a common condition that is on the rise among overweight people. And eating yogurt with live cultures revs up your body's ability to burn fat. A recent study at the University of Tennessee found that people who incorporated yogurt into their diet plan lost 22 percent more weight and 61 percent more body fat than people who simply reduced their caloric intake. This may stem from the fact that yogurt is high in calcium, which is essential for releasing the hormones that break down fat. So how about adding a little "culture" to your life by enjoying some delicious, fat-flushing yogurt?

Recommended Usage

Up to one cup of whole-fat yogurt per day.

Just the Facts

- Americans eat over 300,000 tons of yogurt each year.
- For most people, eating one cup of yogurt a week is enough to keep their intestines colonized with good bacteria.
- Because of the lactase it contains, yogurt is digested three times faster than milk. This makes it well tolerated by people who are lactose intolerant.

Boost the Benefits

- When you're shopping for yogurt, look for a product that is made from organic milk and spells out which live active cultures it contains. The best-quality products have the following five live bacteria: *S. thermophilus, L. bulgaricus, L. acidophilus, L. casei,* and *L. reuteri.*
- Avoid yogurts that contain artificial colors, flavorings, or sweeteners. This includes fruit-filled yogurt, which often contains excess sugar.
- Remember to check the expiration date on yogurt containers to make sure they are fresh.
- Store yogurt in the refrigerator in its original container. If *unopened,* yogurt stays fresh for about one week past the expiration date.

Be a Fat Flush Cook

- Yogurt can become thin and runny if it is mixed or heated too much. For best results, be careful not to stir it excessively or overheat it.
- Use plain yogurt when you're making dips for fruits and vegetables; sauces for meat, fish, and poultry; and dessert toppings.
- For a delicious dip, add chopped cucumber and fresh dill to plain yogurt.
- Give your morning smoothie a calcium boost by adding a dollop of plain yogurt.
- Have yogurt as a snack, dessert, or light meal. Try a healthy yogurt shake or use plain yogurt in place of sour cream.

THINK TWICE!

- *Even if you have a general intolerance for dairy products, you may be able to eat yogurt because the process of making yogurt transforms the lactose in milk into lactic acid. In studies, yogurt with active lactic acid bacteria improved lactose absorption in lactose-intolerant people. If you want to test your response to yogurt, be sure you purchase plain yogurt that contains live active cultures.*

IT'S BEEN SAID . . .

One of my favorite desserts is both elegant and easy. I alternate layers of yogurt and fresh berries in a large wine glass or snifter. I sprinkle ground flax seeds on top for a bit of crunch. I've even served it at dinner parties and people love it!

PEGGY K., GEORGIA

7 Fat Flush Supplements

It is better to prepare and prevent than to repair and repent.

—Anonymous

Leaves, roots, flowers, bark, stems, and seeds. These are the humble sources of the Fat Flush supplements discussed in this chapter. Giving the body a boost with natural herbs and plants is not new. The medicinal benefits of plants have been known for centuries and span all cultures. Herbs have been used throughout history as a means of enhancing health, curing illness, and preventing disease. In fact, many modern over-the-counter and prescription drugs like aspirin, prednisone, and valium are derived or adapted from the powerful active ingredients in plants

In today's world, because of soil depletion, overfarming, synthetic fertilizers, genetic engineering, and hybrid crops, we can't always get all the nutrients we need from foods—no matter how healthy our diet. I believe that certain supplements are crucial to successful weight loss, ongoing weight control, liver support, and bile decongestion. From essential and critical fatty acids to liver-cleansing herbs and redox-signaling molecules, the following Fat Flush supplements are your "support system," extra weapons in your arsenal against inflammation, aging, and weight gain.

Every year, sales of herbal supplements amount to hundreds of millions of dollars in the United States alone. And health food stores and now supermarkets carry a bewildering number of items. How can you know which supplements to buy? It is crucial to purchase only those products that you know to be of superior quality and that are fitting for your particular biochemistry. Otherwise, you may be wasting your money or not getting what is indicated on the label—or you may be getting more, in the way of sugar, additives, fillers, and preservatives.

Many of the herbal supplements available today target specific problems, such as arthritis pain, muscle spasms, or a weak immune system. The focus of the Fat Flush supplements is, of course, to gently support the liver and decongesting bile while promoting fat burning and weight loss—without the use of harmful substances like ephedra or guarana. In addition, these Fat Flush supplements all offer additional benefits that help us in our quest to be strong and vital—now and in the years to come.

ASEA

> ### Fat Flush Factors
>
> *Detoxifier*
> *Energizer*

You probably already know the importance of antioxidants, but there is a new player on the market called ASEA, which boosts the activity of the antioxidants in your body. Your ability to stay healthy and energized relies on how well your cells function, and this in turn depends on something called redox signaling. This communication is responsible for critical messages within and between your cells that coordinate their activities in a way that maximizes your health. Increasing redox signaling molecules can deliver antiaging benefits, enhanced antioxidant activity, improved cellular communication, better immune function, and greater athletic performance.

As we age, our defenses are weakened by stress and environmental toxins. As normal cellular function declines, so does the body's ability to produce and maintain a proper balance of redox signaling molecules. This is where ASEA comes in—it replenishes these molecules.

According to the company, one of the antioxidants ASEA can activate is glutathione, your "master antioxidant." In a study involving overweight and obese women, ASEA reduced oxidative stress, arterial stiffness, and oxidized LDL. Another study showed it to accelerate the rate of cell death (apoptosis)—in a good way, purging your body of sick and damaged cells.

How important are antioxidants in preventing things like type 2 diabetes and heart disease? Very important! We know that fat cells exposed to certain antioxidants produce lower levels of an enzyme that forms triglycerides, and higher triglycerides will increase your risk of heart disease. A recent study found that oxidative stress may be the key trigger in the development of insulin resistance and type 2 diabetes—even more than inflammation.

ASEA is a specially formulated saline solution that you drink. According to the manufacturer, ASEA has been scientifically shown to make positive shifts in serum biomarkers within 30 minutes of drinking it, and these benefits continue to amp up your energy and boost your antioxidant activity for 24 hours. One in vitro study reported that ASEA improved overall antioxidant efficiency by more than 500 percent.

ASEA is a "redox" supplement. Okay . . . so what does this mean? Redox is short for *reduction* and *oxidation*, and the molecules that are responsible for redox signaling operations are absolutely vital to life. Redox signaling is necessary for continued cell production and repair, detoxification, and proper immune function; and your mitochondria—those little powerhouses inside every cell of your body—are central to this process.

Here's a little Science 101 for your inner geek, because it will help you better understand what your body needs to stay healthy. Reduction and oxidation refer to the transfer of electrons (negatively charged particles). When a molecule or atom receives an electron, its electrical charge is reduced—meaning, it becomes more negatively charged. (Remember your basic algebra? $-1 + -1 = -2$.)

Conversely, when a molecule or atom has some of its electrons removed, it's said to be oxidized. Basically, cellular signaling involves these transfers of electrons back and forth between various atoms and molecules in your body.

Redox signaling molecules control this process and fall into two types: reactive oxygen species and reduced species. However, when you hear the term *redox signaling*, it's probably more helpful to think in terms of free radicals and antioxidants.

Free radicals are molecules or atoms that "steal" electrons from other atoms, thereby oxidizing the other. The free radical that gains an electron by stealing it is reduced, and often these bad boys create inflammation and other havoc in the body. Antioxidants help you by neutralizing free radicals. Neutralizing free radicals is also referred to as "reducing oxidative stress."

There ends your redox science lesson—but here's the kicker: regardless of how many antioxidants you ingest, they can't fight free radicals unless they're activated, and ASEA was developed with this in mind. Activating them triggers the cellular communication that's necessary for healing. In fact, the healing response is actually a well-orchestrated effort to repair your damaged cells—or hit their self-destruct buttons so they can be replaced by new and healthy ones. Redox molecules are the conductors of this orchestra. ASEA can be a great adjunct to my New Fat Flush Plan by helping you maximize the antioxidant power from your foods and supplements.

Recommended Usage

ASEA's manufacturer recommends drinking two to four ounces once or twice daily on an empty stomach, with the best results coming from four ounces per serving during the first month.

Just the Facts

- ASEA is made by a company of the same name, which launched the product in 2010. The word *asea* means "by the sea," said to symbolize "rejuvenation, rebirth, and healing" at the cellular level.

Boost the Benefits

- ASEA is not temperature sensitive, and so it does not need to be refrigerated.

THINK TWICE!

- *There are no cautions or known side effects of ASEA.*

CHOLINE

Fat Flush Factors
Cholesterol Zapper
Detoxifier
Energizer

Before 1998, scientists believed that the human body made adequate amounts of choline. However, after additional research, the National Academy of Sciences classified choline as an essential nutrient—and acknowledged that we can't always produce the required amount. More about this later. Unfortunately, coming up short on choline can lead to hypertension, arteriosclerosis, cirrhosis, and fatty deposits in the liver.

Choline is vital to controlling fat and cholesterol buildup in the body; regulating the kidneys, liver, and gallbladder; and banishing fatigue. Recent studies have concluded that choline helps the body burn fat while simultaneously lowering cholesterol. As an added bonus, choline helps form phosphatidylcholine, which is needed for proper mental functioning. Providing your body with adequate choline while you are young can help diminish memory deficits as you age. Choline can nourish your brain *and* your liver while it helps you lose weight. That's quite a deal.

Recommended Usage

Based on current research, a reasonable amount of choline supplementation is 250 to 1,000 milligrams daily. I suggest 300 to 350 milligrams per day.

Just the Facts

- Choline is an essential nutrient sometimes referred to as vitamin B4.
- Just a few weeks on a choline-deficient diet has been shown to cause abnormal liver function.
- The main dietary source of choline is lecithin (also discussed later), which is found in foods such as eggs, fish, and seeds such as sunflower.

Boost the Benefits

- You may want to take choline supplements early in the day, because some people find that choline interferes with their sleep if taken in the evening.
- Taking choline right before a meal is fine, although it works equally well when taken with food.

CHROMIUM

Fat Flush Factors
Blood Sugar Stabilizer *Cholesterol Zapper* *Energizer*

Since the 1960s, researchers have known that chromium plays a vital role in the metabolism of glucose and is needed for proper insulin function and energy production. If we don't get enough chromium, we suffer from impaired insulin activity known as insulin resistance. As the body becomes insulin resistant, more glucose remains in the bloodstream and ends up being stored as fat, rather than moving into the cells to be burned for energy. Chromium helps stabilize blood sugar levels and is also crucial to the synthesis of cholesterol, fats, and proteins. Since overweight people are often insulin resistant, chromium is a natural choice for promoting a healthy metabolism, reducing body fat, and preserving lean muscle.

In fact, chromium is a dieter's dream supplement. It serves to suppress the appetite and reduce cravings. Additionally, it has been shown to build muscle and trim fat at the same time. A recent study, published in *Current Therapeutic Research*, reported on a group of overweight volunteers who were given 400 micrograms of chromium for 72 days. Even though they followed no particular diet or exercise regime, they lost an average of over 4 pounds of fat while gaining 1.4 pounds of lean muscle.

While chromium is found in tiny amounts in many foods, it is difficult to consume enough to meet our needs—especially as we get older. Lifestyle has an impact, as both strenuous exercise and a diet high in sugar cause the body to use chromium more rapidly. To make matters worse, American soil has become chromium deficient. How can you tell if you are lacking in this essential mineral? Some of the symptoms include anxiety, coronary blood vessel disease, depression, diabetes, high cholesterol, hyperinsulinism, hypoglycemia, hyperactivity, and obesity.

Recommended Usage

The Reference Daily Intake for chromium is 120 micrograms, but clinical research suggests that 200 to 400 micrograms is needed for optimal health benefits.

Just the Facts

- The older we get, the less chromium our bodies are able to store.
- When the body is lacking chromium, it takes *twice* as long for insulin to remove glucose from the blood.

Boost the Benefits

- Chromium works best if taken *before* meals.
- Get all the chromium you need by taking the Fat Flush Weight Loss Formula.

THINK TWICE!

- *Don't exceed a daily chromium dose of 1,200 micrograms, because too much chromium may result in liver and kidney problems.*
- *Pregnant or breastfeeding women should avoid chromium supplements.*

IT'S BEEN SAID . . .

I've lost 50 pounds and 30 inches with the help of the Fat Flush Weight Loss Formula, which includes chromium and other fat-burning supplements. The weight loss formula helped me feel full quickly so I never left the table still hungry!

CHRIS P., VIRGINIA

CLA

Fat Flush Factors
Blood Sugar Stabilizer
Energizer

A powerful tool for dieters, CLA, or conjugated linoleic acid, offers profound fat loss and healing benefits. This necessary fatty acid helps reduce body fat while retaining lean muscle mass and is an important building block for cellular growth. Before the 1970s, Americans didn't need to worry about supplementing their diets with CLA since dairy products and meats contained ample amounts naturally. But today, because livestock is no longer grass fed, our intake of CLA has dropped by 80 percent. People who have shied away from eating meat and dairy products because of their fat content have further compounded this deficiency. Fortunately, researchers discovered a way to create CLA from the linoleic acid found in sunflower and safflower oils, and CLA is now available in a convenient capsule form.

Why is CLA such a boon to waist watchers? Study after study has shown its effectiveness in reducing body fat. The *Journal of Nutrition* published the results of the first human clinical trial using CLA, which showed a dramatic 20 percent decrease in body fat, with an average loss of seven pounds of fat in the group taking CLA. These results were achieved without a single change in dietary habits, establishing CLA supplementation as a simple, effortless weight loss tool. Another recent clinical trial, conducted at the University of Wisconsin, assessed the effects of CLA on the body composition of 80 obese men and women. All the participants dieted for several months, lost weight, and then returned to their old eating habits. While the group taking CLA did regain some weight, they put the pounds back on in a ratio of half fat to half lean muscle, compared with 75 percent fat to 25 percent muscle for the control group. This evidence suggests that CLA increases lean muscle mass and results in a stronger, healthier body.

The benefits of CLA do not stop at weight loss. Over the past two decades, researchers have found that CLA also modulates the immune response, protects against heart disease, and inhibits the growth of various cancers. It may also prevent and control adult onset diabetes, a disease running rampant in our overweight country. And because it helps prevent bone loss, CLA may also be a potent agent for preventing osteoporosis and osteoarthritis. The message is clear: along with a balanced diet and a daily exercise program, CLA can help you fight disease and pare off the pounds.

Recommended Usage

Three to six grams daily, taken before or with meals.

Just the Facts

- CLA was first discovered in 1987 by researchers at the University of Wisconsin in Madison.
- CLA permeates muscles cells, where it has been shown to increase muscle mass by as much as 5 percent.
- You'd need to eat 6 pounds of steak or 50 slices of Colby cheese to receive the same amount of conjugated linoleic acid found in most CLA dietary supplement products.

Boost the Benefits

- Occasionally, people find that if they take CLA close to bedtime, they have trouble falling asleep. I recommend that you experiment and see how your body reacts. Most people can take CLA after a late dinner and have no problems sleeping.
- It's best to avoid taking CLA with fiber supplements or high-fiber meals because the fiber may absorb some of the CLA. For best results, take CLA an hour or so after a high-fiber meal or fiber supplements.
- For weight management, most people report noticeable results after taking CLA for about six weeks.

GLA

Fat Flush Factors
Energizer
Thermogenic

Since the 1980s, many studies have focused on the power of GLA, or gamma-linolenic acid, to serve as a natural aid to weight loss. Found naturally in seed oils, such as borage, evening primrose, and black currant seed oils, GLA is an essential fatty acid that triggers fat burning instead of fat storage by boosting the metabolism. It does this in two ways: First, it fuels the burning of brown adipose tissue, a type of fat commonly dormant in overweight people. Second, it stimulates a metabolic process commonly referred to as the "sodium pump," helping to use up nearly half of the body's calories.

In a healthy body, GLA can be synthesized from linoleic acid, which is found in certain oils, grains, and seeds. But because of a number of common dietary and lifestyle factors in today's society, most of our bodies don't make that conversion. The main metabolic roadblocks are artificial trans fats, sugar, smoking, alcohol, aging, and illnesses such as diabetes. All these factors affect the body's ability to convert linoleic acid into GLA and efficiently burn fat.

Luckily, it's easy to give your body the GLA it needs to become an efficient fat-burning machine. As noted above, GLA is found naturally in seed oils like borage oil (20–24 percent GLA), evening primrose oil (8–10 percent GLA), and black currant seed oil (about 15 percent GLA). Supplementing with these oils provides GLA in a usable form, so the body can bypass the conversion process and get down to the business of burning excess fat.

Like other fatty acids, GLA is thought to help to elevate levels of serotonin, a brain chemical that contributes to the feeling of fullness. This is perhaps the reason why you will feel satisfied sooner, which puts the brakes on the urge to overindulge.

The benefits of GLA extend beyond weight loss. It also controls PMS symptoms, lowers high blood pressure, wards off rheumatoid arthritis, and may help certain drug-resistant cancers. And a steady supply of GLA helps skin retain its moisture and stay supple and smooth.

Recommended Usage

The recommended dose of GLA ranges from 300 to 2,000 milligrams per day. I suggest 360 milligrams taken in two daily doses of 180 milligrams each.

Just the Facts

• Medical studies from around the world make it clear that nearly every area of the body can benefit from GLA supplementation.
• Essential fatty acids, including GLA, were "uncovered" by scientists during the 1980s.

Boost the Benefits

• It may take three to six weeks before you feel the full effects of GLA supplementation.
• GLA is most effective when taken in two doses daily.
• Take GLA with food to enhance its absorption and minimize the likelihood of digestive upset.
• Like other polyunsaturated fats, evening primrose, black currant, and borage oils are easily oxidized and can spoil when exposed to heat, light, and oxygen. Even softgels, which are designed to prevent oxidation, can turn rancid. Store them in a cool, dry place away from light.
• Do not cook with GLA oils. They will break down and become ineffective if exposed to high heat.

THINK TWICE!

• *If you take prescription blood thinners, such as warfarin, check with your doctor before taking evening primrose oil. This form of GLA may impair the ability of your blood to clot.*
• *Rancid GLA products often taste or smell "funny" and are more likely to cause digestive upset.*

GREEN POWDER

Fat Flush Factors
Blood Sugar Stabilizer *Cholesterol Zapper* *Detoxifier* *Energizer*

Greens are some of the most nutrient-dense foods on the planet, loaded with essential vitamins and minerals, antioxidants, and other disease-fighting phytonutrients. As a Fat Flush superfood, they also help build a resilient immune system, nourish and cleanse your blood, and build strong bones, teeth, hair, and nails.

Since so many of us cannot get in all of our daily green veggies on the go, powdered supergreens are an excellent way to enjoy more green vegetables in your diet. Many green powders have appeared on the market of late, but they're not all created equal in terms of quality and purity. From a clean source, however, a green powder can really kick up your nutritional intake several notches—tossing a scoop into your morning smoothie can skyrocket your energy level for the entire day

Green powders are only as powerful as the individual vegetables they contain, and each veggie has its own complement of nutrients and therefore its own unique set of benefits. I have my favorites of course—take barley grass, for example. Barley grass repairs DNA twice as fast chlorophyll, protects you from free-radical damage, and can boost your brain power—in addition to providing many other health benefits.

Broccoli is another superstar veggie, and broccoli sprouts are like broccoli on steroids! Broccoli sprouts fight *H. pylori* bacteria to prevent and heal ulcers, optimize lipids and blood pressure, reduce insulin resistance, and assist with DNA repair. They're a rich source of sulforaphane, a cancer-preventative compound. This small molecule enters human cells with ease, behaving as a "signaling molecule" to communicate with other cells. Potentially affecting more than 2,000 genes and activating multiple defense mechanisms, sulforaphane allows your body to reprogram its DNA into peak performance.

Another of my favorite greens is chlorella, which supports your immune, digestive, and cardiovascular systems, as well as helping with detoxification. It's high in beta-carotene, vitamin D, and gamma-linolenic acid and provides the nine essential amino acids.

One veggie you will seldom find in green powders is celery, but it's an underappreciated addition! As a formulator and spokesperson for Uni Key Health Systems, Inc., I insisted that celery be added to the greens blend because it's a naturally rich source of bioavailable vegetable sodium. This type of sodium acts like an adaptogen and blood pressure stabilizer. Celery protects the digestive tract and liver and helps heal stomach ulcers. It's also a crucial nutrient for tired adrenal glands, helping you cope more effectively with mental, emotional, and physiological stress.

Don't forget about bitter greens—the more you can squeeze into your daily diet the better, so look for a green powder that has some in the mix. Bitter greens such as dandelion, arugula, kale, and collards help build your bile and turn your liver into a fat-burning and cleansing machine. Superrich in magnesium, kale and collards help reduce blood pressure and soothe anxiety. Collards support immune regulation and have antibacterial and antiviral properties to boot. My other favorite super-greens include alfalfa grass, wheat grass, oat grass, parsley, and spinach. Wheat grass, by the way, is generally considered gluten-free and can be tolerated by the gluten sensitive.

One word of caution: green powders can be heavily contaminated. Just as they concentrate nutrients, if they are not made from clean sources, they can concentrate toxins, including heavy metals. This is especially true of sea vegetables, which can be repositories of not only heavy metals but radiation residues. (That's why for Uni Key's Daily Greens I chose chlorella that was specially grown under monitored conditions.)

Research shows that greens can support detoxification—but of course this isn't possible if your greens are full of toxins themselves. In 2013, ConsumerLab performed testing on 11 different "greens" and "whole-foods" products, finding five contaminated with lead, arsenic, and bacteria. So you must choose your green powder wisely.

Recommended Usage

- Many green powders are tasty all by themselves, so you can just mix them into water and drink up. The flavor is a little like tea.
- Add a scoop of greens to your daily smoothie or stir into a glass of nut milk, tigernut milk, or coconut milk.
- Make "green eggs and ham," maybe minus the ham . . . got the picture?
- Add a little to your bowl of oatmeal, as long as you don't mind a green hue.
- Give your soup a scoop!
- Add to cake or brownie batter—just make sure you are using a healthful brownie recipe to begin with.
- Knead it into your burger or sausage.

- You can augment the flavor and health benefits of green drinks by adding a pinch or two of Celtic Sea Salt, which provides dozens of important trace minerals.

Boost the Benefits

- Ideally, you want a green powder that is cold processed, and top-quality varieties are freeze-dried. One source reports that 80 percent of the green powders on the market today are heat processed.
- Choose a green powder with non-GMO, preferably organic ingredients.
- Avoid any that contain fructose or fruit juice concentrates, which are a hidden source of fructose. Fructose places stress on your liver and is linked to nonalcoholic fatty liver disease (NAFLD), weight gain, and high LDL levels, which increase your cardiovascular risk.
- You may want to avoid formulas that incorporate sea vegetables. Although sea vegetables such as kelp and spirulina may be high in trace minerals and micronutrients, they are also notoriously tainted with radioactive residues and heavy metals like lead, cadmium, mercury, and arsenic.
- Choose powdered greens that easily dissolve in water, juice, or other beverages.

THINK TWICE!

- *As mentioned earlier, be careful about the source of your product and how it's made. Make sure you're buying a green powder that uses pristine sources.*

Fat Flush Fun

- Perhaps the earliest example of a "green powder" is matcha, which dates back to the Tang Dynasty (seventh- to tenth-century China). Matcha is a powdered green tea you mix with hot water, very high in antioxidants and cancer-fighting phytochemicals.

IT'S BEEN SAID . . .

A green powder supplement is like a multivitamin on steroids.

NUTRITIONIST TERESA BOYCE

LECITHIN

Fat Flush Factors

Blood Sugar Stabilizer
Cholesterol Zapper
Detoxifier

Adding a tablespoon of lecithin to your smoothie is like adding detergent to your dishwater—it melts fat off your hips and thighs, breaking it down so your body can use what it needs and flush the rest away. This underappreciated fat-melting food deserves much more attention than it gets!

But what *is* lecithin? It's a naturally occurring fatty compound found in plant and animal tissues, a vital component of every cell that helps keep cell membranes nourished, pliable, and healthy. Lecithin makes up about 30 percent of your brain, as well as two-thirds of the myelin sheaths surrounding your brain, nerves, and spinal cord. There is evidence that multiple sclerosis sufferers are deficient in lecithin, which makes sense when you consider MS is a disease of the myelin sheaths.

Lecithin is made up of choline (as mentioned earlier), fatty acids, glycerol, glycolipids, phospholipids, phosphoric acid, and triglycerides. It serves as a fat emulsifier, breaking down and dispersing fats in order to increase their bioavailability. Your liver produces lecithin when it has adequate building blocks, but often these nutritional components are in short supply.

Among other things, your body breaks down lecithin into choline, a precursor to the very important nerve transmitter acetylcholine. Acetylcholine is a chemical messenger responsible for keeping your heart beating and activating your muscles and glands and is also responsible for peristalsis and learning and memory. It was the first neurotransmitter ever discovered—and the most abundant.

Ninety percent of us do not receive enough choline. Choline plays numerous roles in your liver, brain, muscles, nervous system, and overall metabolism, including synthesizing DNA and carrying cholesterol away from the liver. Choline requirements rise exponentially for pregnant women because it's critical for fetal development. Choline plays a key role in methylation as well, which is vital to nearly every biological process. Understanding methylation is complicated, but basically it involves the transfer of methyl groups. Your diet is a major source of choline, and organic pastured eggs are one of the best sources. In fact, lecithin was first isolated from egg yolks.

Lecithin has evidence-based benefits for Alzheimer's and other forms of dementia as well as for anxiety, eczema, liver and gallbladder problems, immune function, and your heart. It has profound benefits for your liver and gallbladder because it helps build and thin the bile, keeping it flowing freely and preventing blockages. Choline helps regenerate the part of your liver that makes bile. Lecithin helps break down fats so they can more easily be digested. Because lecithin emulsifies fat, it helps prevent and dissolve gallstones—which are basically calcified fat gravel!

Between 66 percent and 75 percent of your liver contains lecithin to break down fats. When lecithin is diminished, fats will not be properly excreted and will build up, which not only accumulates in your midsection but also results in nonalcoholic fatty liver disease. NAFLD can lead to more serious conditions such as type 2 diabetes, cirrhosis, and even liver cancer. Lecithin is also necessary for proper absorption of fat-soluble vitamins A, D, E, and K and can protect from the damage by hepatitis and alcohol-related cirrhosis.

Lecithin has also been shown to benefit your heart. Lecithin supplementation can reduce hyperlipidemia, improve lipid metabolism, break up plaques, and help reverse atherosclerosis. In a 2010 study involving individuals with suboptimal lipid profiles, 500 milligrams of soy lecithin daily reduced LDL levels by an astonishing 42 percent after one month of treatment and 56 percent after two months.

Lecithin also helps keep homocysteine levels low. Choline is involved in the methylation of homocysteine into methionine, so when choline is low, homocysteine levels rise, along with your risk for cardiovascular disease. Choline tamps down inflammation.

Lecithin is neuroprotective in part because of its antioxidant actions, which have been compared to those of alpha-tocopherol (vitamin E). One of lecithin's compounds is phosphatidylserine, a phospholipid that dampens your stress response. The choline in lecithin is known to reduce anxiety, as well as reducing manic symptoms associated with bipolar disorder. Adults age 50 to 85 receiving 1,000 milligrams of choline daily showed improvements in brain function in terms of memory and processing. Even your immune system may get a jump start from lecithin—scientists found that it stimulated macrophage and lymphocyte activity in rats.

Taking a lecithin supplement is an easy and effective way to boost your body's lecithin stores. Supplements can be purchased as liquid, granules, or capsules. Today, lecithin is regularly extracted from cottonseed, marine sources, milk, rapeseed, soybeans, and sunflower seeds—but soy and sunflower are by far the most common.

With the prevalence of GMOs today, make sure you avoid conventional soy lecithin and opt for organic non-GMO. Be aware that soy lecithin contains trace amounts of soy proteins, and although those may include minute amounts of soy allergens, the residues appear to be insufficient to provoke allergic reactions in the majority of the soy-sensitive individuals.

A few companies are now offering sunflower lecithin, which is a good option if you want to avoid soy altogether. Advantages of sunflower lecithin are reported to be a healthier extraction process—typically cold processed without the use of solvents such as acetone and hexane, which are often used to extract lecithin from soybeans. Sunflower lecithin is even available raw. You'll have to weigh the pros and cons for yourself. Most of the research studies have been based on soy lecithin.

Recommended Usage

- Blend a tablespoon or two into your morning smoothie. Lecithin generally thickens anything it's added to.
- Liquid lecithin is more concentrated than granules, so you only need about half.
- Lecithin can take the place of eggs in recipes that require emulsification. In many recipes, lecithin can be substituted in equal parts for oil or butter. Add it to gluten-free baked goods to improve texture and cohesion.
- Try adding it to sauces, gravies, soups, nut butters, nut milks, and even salad dressings for a creamy, homogenous texture.
- Add it to meatballs for cohesion, as an alternative to eggs.

Just the Facts

- The word *lecithin* comes from the Greek term *lekythos*, which means "egg yolk." In 1846, Gobley isolated lecithin from egg yolk and in 1850 gave it its present name.
- Vegans are more susceptible to lecithin-choline deficiency, since the richest sources are animal products (seafood, fish, poultry, meat, organ meats, etc.). Vegetable sources include collard greens, cauliflower, broccoli, cabbage, and bok choy.

Boost the Benefits

- Make sure you choose organic non-GMO lecithin, as more than 90 percent of soybeans are genetically engineered today.

THINK TWICE!

- In some people, lecithin has been reported to cause bloating, nausea, stomach pain, diarrhea, or mild skin rash. If you have soy allergies, you may want to avoid soy lecithin.

IT'S BEEN SAID . . .

Two tablespoons per day makes the fat go away.

Or how about:

Two tablespoons a day keeps the gallstones away.

L-METHIONINE

Fat Flush Factors

Cholesterol Zapper
Detoxifier
Thermogenic

An essential amino acid, L-methionine teams up in your body with choline and inositol to form a powerful trio of nutrients that assists in the breakdown of fats. L-methionine helps lower cholesterol levels by increasing the liver's production of lecithin. At the same time, it prevents excess fat buildup in the liver and is an excellent detoxifier, ridding the body of heavy metals such as lead, cadmium, and mercury.

Through its supply of sulfur, L-methionine protects cells from airborne toxins, such as smog. This helps prevent disorders of the hair, skin, and nails, all the while slowing down the aging process. This little amino acid also protects the kidneys by creating ammonia-free urine. In a recent study of women with recurring urinary tract infections, L-methionine was found to prevent bacteria from adhering to the cells of the urinary tract, thereby sparing the women from yet another bladder infection.

Because the body can't produce L-methionine, we have to get it from food or supplements. To ensure adequate daily amounts, I recommend supplementation.

Recommended Usage

A supplement of 100 milligrams per day.

Just the Facts

- Small daily amounts of methionine are enough for most people to maintain good health.
- L-methionine can be found in meat, eggs, onions, beans, lentils, and yogurt.

Boost the Benefits

• You'll benefit most from L-methionine if you take it before meals.
• L-methionine is most effective when your body has an adequate supply of magnesium, so be sure you're getting at least 400 milligrams of magnesium per day.

THINK TWICE!

• *Studies have shown that cancer patients should not take L-methionine because of its tendency to feed tumors.*

MAGNESIUM

Fat Flush Factors
Blood Sugar Stabilizer
Cholesterol Zapper
Detoxifier

If there is a superstar of the mineral kingdom, it's magnesium. Magnesium is the "master mineral" for more than 300 key metabolic operations. Scientists have detected 3,751 magnesium-binding sites on human proteins, suggesting that its role in health and disease has been vastly underappreciated. Magnesium is the only mineral whose deficiency is linked to all of the Big Four: cancer, stroke, heart disease, and diabetes.

The fact that 80 percent of Americans are deficient in this extremely important mineral is a very serious public health problem!

A century of science has uncovered the links between magnesium deficiency and everything from type 2 diabetes to chronic fatigue and fibromyalgia, migraines, dementia, and osteoporosis. Early signs of deficiency are varied but include problems like insomnia, irritability, depression, loss of appetite, headache, facial twitches, nausea, fatigue, and weakness, to name just a few. One of magnesium's major functions is pulling back the reins on inflammation. If your magnesium levels fall, you get a massive bounce in inflammatory cytokines and histamines, and all of that spells pain and increased risk for multiple chronic illnesses, including the Big Four already mentioned.

Magnesium is clearly linked to cardiovascular risk. The more magnesium you have in your body, the lower your chances for heart attack and stroke. This megamineral may even lower your risk for cancer. A meta-analysis published in the *American Journal of Clinical Nutrition* found that those with higher magnesium intake enjoyed a lower risk for colorectal tumors.

If you're struggling with weight issues, blood sugar instability, or food cravings, take a look at your magnesium intake. Several studies have highlighted magnesium's role in revving up your metabolism—specifically in terms of insulin sensitivity, glucose regulation, and protection from type 2 diabetes. Magnesium also improves digestion, discourages kidney stone formation, and is a primo detox mineral to boot!

Magnesium helps activate your muscles and nerves and helps your body make ATP for energy. Higher intake is associated with higher bone density in both men and women. Magnesium also serves as a precursor for neurotransmitters with associated benefits for depression, anxiety, and attention disorders. Additionally, magnesium has proven benefits for migraine sufferers.

Your body requires about 500 to 1,000 milligrams of magnesium daily, and the average American takes in less than half. Only 1 percent of the magnesium in your body is distributed in your blood, making blood tests only marginally useful for detecting deficiencies. Most magnesium is stored in your bones and organs. Dietary magnesium is immediately used to deal with everyday mental and physical stresses related to food allergies and intolerances, prescription drugs, heavy-metal exposure, and other environmental insults. Magnesium is an adaptogenic mineral and is simply "used up" faster than many can replace it.

Factors that can further deplete magnesium stores include high levels of stress, suboptimal digestive function, excessive alcohol or soda intake, caffeine, and aging in general—meaning that we generally need more as we age.

Bottom line: the vast majority of us would benefit from a high-quality magnesium supplement. There are a wide variety of supplements on the market because the mineral must be bound to another substance—there is no such thing as a 100 percent magnesium supplement. Unfortunately, the most popular cofactors used are oxide and citrate, and these primarily target your gut and act as laxatives, making a good deal typically lost through the bowel.

The latest research shows that there are better options for supporting our overstressed hearts and overworked brains. Glycinate, malate, taurate, and orotate are the best forms of magnesium for head-to-toe health and are more bioavailable than other forms. Additionally, it's important that you get enough calcium and vitamins B6, K2, and D, because they work synergistically with magnesium in your body. Vitamin B6 is particularly notable, as it determines how much magnesium will be absorbed by your cells. Also realize that low magnesium (not just low calcium) can prevent your body from properly utilizing your vitamin D.

Recommended Usage

- Not sure which form of magnesium is best for you? Ideally, take a supplement with a combination of several forms, because different forms have different functions in your body.
- For insomnia, anxiety, moodiness, or stress, try magnesium glycinate.
- To boost heart health and prevent migraines, take magnesium taurate (magnesium combined with the amino acid taurine).
- Magnesium orotate also helps repair the heart, as well as boosting athletic performance and DNA repair.

- For improving energy and muscle function or for treating digestive issues, PMS, or fibromyalgia, magnesium malate is your best friend. Magnesium malate is a combination of magnesium and malic acid.
- Magnesium oxide and magnesium citrate primarily target the gut and so are useful as laxatives—which is why mag citrate is prescribed to clean out the colon before people undergo some medical procedures (think colonoscopy).

Just the Facts

- Magnesium is depleted by today's commercial farming methods much more than calcium.
- Magnesium prevents the formation of kidney stones by inhibiting the binding of calcium with oxalate, the two compounds of which they're composed.
- Muscle cramps or insomnia can be a sign of magnesium deficiency.
- Tinnitus (a constant, high-pitched ringing in the ears) and hearing loss may also be symptoms of magnesium deficiency.

Boost the Benefits

- Diet is the absolute best source of any mineral, and magnesium is no exception. The best foods to shore up your magnesium stores are dark green leafy veggies, seaweed (especially kelp and dulse), almonds and cashews, beets, and bananas.
- Here's a news flash to lift your spirits: dark chocolate contains a substantial dose of magnesium—95 milligrams per one square. That's more mag than an ounce of almonds, one-eighth cup of pumpkin seeds, or two-thirds cup of spinach or chard!
- The average cup of coffee contains about seven grams of magnesium.
- Keep in mind that there are additional ways to increase your magnesium. You can use topical magnesium oil or take an Epsom salt bath, which is magnesium sulfate. Try rubbing magnesium oil on the bottoms of your feet at night before going to bed for a deep, relaxing slumber.

Fat Flush in Action

- Replace your ordinary table salt with natural sea salt, which is rich in natural minerals including magnesium.

THINK TWICE!

- *Oral magnesium toxicity is uncommon, because your body eliminates excess amounts through the bowel, unless you have serious problems with your kidneys. Ordinarily, you'll know you're taking too much magnesium if you develop diarrhea because of magnesium's laxative effects. Diarrhea is more common with magnesium citrate and magnesium oxide.*

Fat Flush Fun

- Magnesium is named for the Greek city of Magnesia, a source of calcium oxide, also called magnesia.
- Magnesium is the eleventh-most abundant element in the human body, the third-most abundant mineral in seawater, and the eighth-most abundant element in the entire universe.
- Magnesium is formed in large stars (only those with a mass of eight or more Earth suns) by fusing helium with neon.
- A magnesium ion lies at the center of every chlorophyll molecule in every green plant.

IT'S BEEN SAID . . .

I heard that oxygen and magnesium were going out and I was like O-Mg.

MILK THISTLE

Fat Flush Factors
Detoxifier

Did you know that weight gain, cellulite, and abdominal bloating are just a few of the signs that the liver is overburdened? It's true. When your liver is sluggish, every organ in your body is affected, and your weight loss efforts are blocked. Some common reasons why the liver gets overloaded include environmental toxins, processed foods, overeating, and damaging factors such as alcohol, contraceptive pills, candida, and caffeine.

But there's good news! One of the world's most thoroughly studied herbs, milk thistle, is a powerful antioxidant that has been shown to support detoxification of the liver, speed up liver function, and help regenerate new, healthy liver cells. It also changes the makeup of bile, helping to reduce the risk of gallstones.

A member of the sunflower family, milk thistle gets its strength from a complex compound called silymarin, which scavenges free radicals and inhibits free-radical production. Silymarin defends the liver against toxins by changing the structure of liver cells so that toxins can't get in, thereby protecting and curing the liver at the same time. So support your liver and improve your chances to lose weight with a daily dose of milk thistle.

Recommended Usage

Take 200 milligrams per day.

Just the Facts

- Milk thistle has been used medicinally for more than 2,000 years and has been the subject of clinical trials for over 40 years.
- It is not uncommon to find milk thistle growing wild in a variety of settings, including by the side of the road. (But you should "harvest" your milk thistle in the form of a quality supplement.)

Boost the Benefits

- Although milk thistle is available as a tea, you're better off taking it in capsule or tablet form. Milk thistle is not particularly water soluble, so steeping it in a tea diminishes its liver-protective benefits.

- While milk thistle may be purchased as a "stand-alone" supplement, it is absorbed better when combined with choline. You may purchase the two separately and take them at the same time, or you may find a supplement that combines the two.

THINK TWICE!

- *Since milk thistle boosts liver and gallbladder activity, it may have a mild laxative effect in some people. This usually lasts for only two to three days.*

OREGON GRAPE ROOT

Fat Flush Factors
Cholesterol Zapper
Detoxifier
Energizer

Oregon grape is a tall shrub native to the western regions of Canada and the United States. Early American physicians learned about the medicinal benefits of Oregon grape root from the Native Americans, who used it to cure a number of ailments. Now scientists know that it is the berberine in Oregon grape root that prevents infections by boosting the immune system and destroying bacteria. The grape root purifies the blood by activating infection-fighting blood cells known as macrophages.

In addition, Oregon grape root stimulates the liver, gallbladder, and thyroid gland. Long known as a "liver tonic," grape root enhances the flow of bile through the liver and gallbladder, helping the liver filter out toxins effectively. However, the benefits of grape root don't stop there. It is also used to treat parasites, arthritis, menstrual cramps, skin diseases, and digestive problems. And because of its energizing effect on the thyroid gland, Oregon grape root fights overall fatigue, thereby helping people regain a youthful vitality.

Recommended Usage

I recommend 200 milligrams daily.

Just the Facts

- Holly-leaf barberry is another name for Oregon grape.
- Oregon grape root contains anticancer compounds called dehydropodophyllotoxin and podophyllotoxin.

THINK TWICE!

- Oregon grape root is not recommended for use during pregnancy and lactation.
- The effectiveness of certain medications, such as doxycycline and tetracycline, may be lessened when taken at the same time as grape root.
- High doses of Oregon grape root may interfere with B vitamin metabolism.

OX BILE

Fat Flush Factors
Blood Sugar Stabilizer
Cholesterol Zapper
Detoxifier

Just as the name implies, ox bile is bile obtained from oxen, typically cows. Because ox bile is made from the bile of an animal, its chemical makeup is similar to our own, so our bodies can use it for the same purpose— specifically, to support fat digestion. Ox bile is helpful for those with low bile production or individuals who've had their gallbladders removed.

Often combined with digestive enzymes such as lipase, protease, and amylase, ox bile is commonly used to treat a number of liver diseases including cirrhosis, hepatitis, Crohn's disease, irritable bowel syndrome (IBS), and short bowel syndrome. However, even if you have no major disease, ox bile can be quite therapeutic.

Bile's critical role in digestion and detoxification is often overlooked, but it is something you truly can't live without. Bile contains bile salts and bile acids, cholesterol esters, and lecithin. Deficiency is very common among adults over 60, especially women—even if you still have your gallbladder. Bile deficiency, or bile that becomes thick and "sludgy," can lead to impaired fat digestion, gallstones, constipation, nutrient malabsorption (especially fat-soluble vitamins A, D, E, and K and essential fatty acids), imbalanced lipid profile, fat accumulation, and weight gain.

Bile acids have multiple functions such as increasing the metabolic activity of brown fat, flushing little gallstones out of your liver, improving insulin sensitivity, stimulating the production of active thyroid hormone in fat cells, and absorbing nutrients. The liver is the body's primary toxin filter, and it sends most of these toxins into the bile to be neutralized. Bile breaks down the walls of viruses and other substances in your gastrointestinal tract.

The latest research also shows that bile acids trigger regeneration in damaged areas of the liver. Cirrhosis occurs when the liver stops regenerating its tissues, replacing them instead with scar tissue, and this impedes the liver's ability to perform any of its normal functions, including production of bile.

How do gallbladder problems and sluggish bile lead to weight gain? Bile is responsible for breaking down fats so they can be used for fuel, instead of as padding for your hips and thighs. And bile requires the assistance of your gallbladder. The gallbladder is a muscular pear-shaped organ sitting just under your liver. Your liver produces about 1 to 1½ quarts of bile per day, which it makes from cholesterol. Your liver sends bile to your gallbladder for storage and concentration.

Adding bile to the food in your gut is like adding soap to your dishwater—it breaks down and disperses (emulsifies) the fat. When fats pass from your stomach into your intestine, your gallbladder receives a message to release bile, which prepares those fats for further processing by the pancreatic enzyme lipase. Once bile is used up, your liver must make more of it, and because it uses cholesterol for this, bile production helps normalize cholesterol levels.

Now for the part that hurts your waistline: When bile is insufficient or sluggish, oversized fat globules make their way into your bloodstream. Because they're not properly broken down, your body cannot use them for fuel, and so they get stored as body fat.

If you've had your gallbladder removed, building up your bile is even *more* important. Gallbladder removal is one of the most common surgeries in the United States today with more than 500,000 performed every year. Without a gallbladder to contain it, bile continuously trickles into your intestine, regardless of when or what you eat. Then, when you do consume a fatty meal, there is no reserve, and over time this not only can result in packing on the pounds, but can cause nutritional deficiencies and other health problems.

Recommended Usage

Use the dosage on the label of your ox bile supplement as a guide. A typical dose is generally about 100 milligrams with each meal, especially fatty meals.

Just the Facts

- Ox, dog, and carp bile have been used for more than a thousand years in Chinese medicine.
- Because bile insufficiency decreases intestinal motility and absorption of nutrients in the colon, ox bile can be helpful for constipation.
- Bile from cows is processed into supplements in a four-step process: extracting, sterilizing, drying (dehydrating), and then crushing into a powder.
- Vegans and vegetarians are often reluctant to use ox bile. Unfortunately, they often have sluggish gallbladders and are in great need of additional bile acids. This is because many vegan-type diets

are low in fat, as well as relatively high in fiber—a combination that can result in bile insufficiency. Fiber tends to bind with bile salts in the intestine, causing them to be excreted rather than reabsorbed, and insufficient dietary fats promote gallbladder sluggishness.

• In 2015, a physician in India removed what was thought to be a new world record for the number of gallstones extracted during one gall-bladder surgery: 11,950 stones! It took medical staff four hours to count the stones, which ranged from 2 to 5 millimeters in size. The patient had been suffering from chronic abdominal pain and acid reflux for two months.

THINK TWICE!

• *The most common side effect of ox bile is diarrhea and occasionally nausea, although this usually only results from too high a dose. Unabsorbed bile salts can have a laxative effect, drawing water into the intestines and causing diarrhea. If this happens, adjust your dose down accordingly. Be particularly careful to start with a low dose if you have any major intestinal issues such as Crohn's or IBS.*

IT'S BEEN SAID . . .

The metaphysical interpretation of sluggish bile and gallstones is bitterness, "hard thoughts," condemnation, pride, resentment, feeling locked in, trying to please others but feeling bitter about it. The liver is said to be the organ where anger is "stored."

TAURINE

Fat Flush Factors
Blood Sugar Stabilizer
Cholesterol Zapper
Detoxifier
Diuretic

Many of us are deficient in taurine. Taurine performs multiple tasks in the body from conjugating bile, to boosting insulin response, to maintaining good cardiac function. Our bodies manufacture taurine from the amino acids cysteine and methionine—but probably not enough for optimal health. Populations with the highest longevity, such as the Japanese, have the highest dietary taurine intake.

We derive sulfur-rich taurine mostly from animal products, but we don't usually consume enough, so our bodies have to manufacture more. As we age, this ability to synthesize taurine gradually declines, making supplementation beneficial.

A common misconception is that taurine is an amino acid, but really it's not—it's technically an amino sulphonic acid, which is a bit different. Nevertheless, taurine is a very important nutrient present in significant amounts throughout the body, particularly in tissues containing excitable cells such as nerves and heart muscle, and it has far-reaching effects. Your body was dependent on taurine even before you were born.

The developing brains of newborns and babies in utero depend on taurine, and they cannot make it for themselves. Taurine deficiency in moms can result in developmental abnormalities, so pregnant and nursing moms—you need to keep your levels up! At least two studies have identified significant taurine deficiencies in autistic children. Taurine's neural effects are not fully understood. It appears to activate GABA receptors in the thalamus, which exert a calming effect. Taurine has been shown to benefit individuals with seizure disorders.

Taurine is also a constituent of bile, encouraging the production of bile acids and thinning of the bile, which is beneficial. It helps prevent nonalcoholic fatty liver disease by removing fat deposits and reducing cirrhosis. Taurine also protects your kidneys from oxidative damage and gives your metabolism a boost by increasing the actions of insulin, stabilizing blood sugar, optimizing lipids, and improving both fat burning and muscle building. Obesity itself has been found to cause a decline in taurine levels, creating a vicious cycle.

Taurine has an abundance of benefits for your heart! It reduces apolipoprotein B100 (apoB), a major component of LDL and VLDL, which increase your risk for atherosclerosis. Taurine also lowers blood pressure, strengthens cardiac output, regulates heartbeat, and protects your heart cells from damage. Animal studies show that for those in congestive heart failure, taurine may reduce mortality by a whopping 80 percent.

Yet another function is keeping your electrolytes in balance (sodium, potassium, magnesium, calcium, and other minerals). Taurine acts like a diuretic, keeping potassium and magnesium inside your cells and excess sodium out. It also regulates the flow of calcium ions, which protects your vision and hearing. Taurine supplementation may lower your risk for macular degeneration and other retinal diseases, tinnitus, and hearing loss. It also plays a role in white blood cell production and bone regeneration.

Recommended Usage

- Incorporate high-quality meats into your diet such as pastured beef and bison, wild game, liver and other organ meats, poultry, fish and shellfish, and pastured eggs. If you are vegan, you can obtain some taurine from seaweed and brewer's yeast, but you will likely need a good daily supplement. Taurine levels are notoriously low among vegans and vegetarians.

Just the Facts

- Taurine was named after the Latin word *taurus*, which means "bull" or "ox," after German scientists first isolated it from ox bile in 1827.
- Certain pathogens can create or exacerbate taurine deficiency. For example, certain anaerobic bacteria degrade taurine. Candida, a systemic fungus, produces the amino acid beta-alanine that competes with taurine for reabsorption by your kidneys and causes loss of taurine in the urine.
- Taurine is degraded by monosodium glutamate.
- Have you ever wondered why taurine is added to commercial cat foods? Unlike dogs and humans, cats cannot make their own taurine, so cat food manufacturers must add it. Despite this, commercial cat foods still tend to be low in taurine due to an overabundance of added starches and low "real meat" content. Taurine deficiency in kitties causes retinal damage and blindness, as well as life-threatening heart problems, including cardiomyopathy.

Boost the Benefits

• Although they often have added taurine, so-called energy drinks are the last place you should think about getting supplemental taurine, as they often also contain large amounts of caffeine, sugar, and toxic chemical additives. The taurine in energy drinks may be at least partly responsible for the "energy crash" experienced by many shortly after consuming them.

THINK TWICE!

• *Interestingly, exposure to sunlight (and other full-spectrum lighting) can increase your body's taurine levels. Those who live or work under fluorescent lighting, which is not full spectrum, may develop taurine deficiency in their pineal and pituitary glands. Over time, this may cause impaired vision.*

IT'S BEEN SAID . . .

Considering its broad distribution, its many cytoprotective attributes, and its functional significance in cell development, nutrition, and survival, . . . taurine is undoubtedly one of the most essential substances in the body.

HARRIS RIPPS AND WEN SHEN,
"REVIEW: TAURINE: A 'VERY ESSENTIAL' AMINO ACID"

8   Fat Flush on a Budget

Eat . . . and be healthy.

—MY GRANDMOTHER CLARA

As we all know only too well, prepackaged, processed foods tend to be easier on the wallet than fresh produce and lean cuts of meat. Unfortunately, those inexpensive "convenience" foods provide little in the way of nutrition, are often high in carbohydrates and calories, and contain a host of unwelcome artificial ingredients.

The good news is that with a little bit of foresight, it is possible to eat nutritious, Fat Flush meals on a budget. I've compiled a variety of tips and practical suggestions for saving money at the supermarket while still providing your body with the healing and slimming superfoods it deserves.

GENERAL TIPS

- Don't go for bulk. Sure, it may be enticing to pick up highly perishable berries when they are on sale, but what a waste if you end up throwing out a whole carton!
- Do make it a rule to stock up on those staples that you can store for a long time. In the freezer, you can safely freeze soup for about two to three months. You can freeze seeds, nuts, nut flours, and seafood for up to a year. In the fridge, you can store eggs for three weeks and flaxseed oil for three months after it is opened. Coconut oil can be stored in the pantry as can olive oil. The same goes for beans, oatmeal, and quinoa as long as your pantry is cool and dry. Stockpile cranberry juice or cranberry concentrate in the pantry when it is on sale and keep all herbs and spices for seasoning away from heat, air, and light.
- Revive the tired veggies you forgot at the bottom of the fridge by soaking in a bath of ice-cold water for a good five minutes or so. Arugula, kale, spinach, and all types of lettuces lend themselves well to this trick. They will be revived quite nicely if you simply dry them off well and then use them in a salad, soup, stir-fry, or even on top of a pizza. You can even pop a variety of tired-looking veggies on a baking sheet and bake them in the oven. They will develop a delicious taste when

they caramelize and can be a respectable side to any protein entrée from poultry to fish to make a complete meal.

• Got leftover herbs, pesto, or sauce? Simply make them into single-serve portions by freezing them in an ice-cube tray. You can add them frozen into any hot soup, sauté, pasta dish, or stir-fry.

• Best to get in the habit of planning a weekly menu. This requires you to have foods on hand, causing you to make fewer trips to the grocery store. Planning also helps you make good use of leftovers, slashing both your cooking time and food costs.

• Avoid shopping for food on an empty stomach. Hungry shoppers buy more than they need.

• To keep from having to discard spoiled produce, use this book as a guide for knowing how long each food may be stored.

• Label foods with the date of purchase *before* you put them away.

• Stop buying junk food and soda. On top of being unhealthy, these items can really take a bite out of your food budget.

• Last, but not least, do what I have done for years—clean your fruits, veggies, eggs, and meats with the Chemist's Formula (see below), and they'll stay fresh for much longer. In addition to avoiding toxic chemicals, you'll stop that expensive practice of throwing out overripe produce.

THE CHEMIST'S FORMULA

This recipe makes one quart of soak that should be prepared fresh each day. The ingredients are 18 drops of grapefruit seed extract with 4 ounces of 3 percent hydrogen peroxide and 1 teaspoon of baking soda per quart. Blend and soak all produce (you can soak eggs as well) for at least 15 minutes; then rinse well, at least three times.

FAT FLUSH STAPLES

• Stock up on cranberries during the fall when they are plentiful in grocery stores. Store them in your freezer and make your own cranberry juice as needed.

• If fresh lemons are expensive in your area, it's fine to use bottled lemon juice. My favorite is the lemon (or lime) juice by Santa Cruz.

• Consider installing a "built-in" ceramic water filter under your sink. While you'll incur an initial cost, you'll pocket significant savings by drinking your own filtered water rather than expensive bottled water.

IT'S BEEN SAID . . .

It's obvious that there are other Fat Flushers in my area because many times, when I'd go shopping for cranberry juice, the shelves at the store would be empty! I'd have to waste time going to other supermarkets and *would often end up buying a different brand of juice that costs $2 more a bottle. Finally, I got smart. I asked my local store to order two cases of cranberry juice for me and asked for a discount. It worked! I order two cases every three months and the store gives me a 10% discount!*

ELLEN H., NORTH CAROLINA

PROTEIN
- Buy "family-size" packages of meat, divide the meat into single servings, and freeze. You'll save money and always have some healthy protein handy.
- To save up to 50 percent on the cost of meat, learn to cut up chickens, bone meat, and grind your own hamburger.

VEGETABLES
- To add zest to grilled foods, save the loose skin on onions and garlic to toss them into the fire just before cooking meats or vegetables.
- Avoid buying produce at convenience stores because you will pay dearly for that "convenience." For example, you'll pay double the price for the "quick stop" cucumber than you would for the same vegetable at the supermarket.
- Make Fat Flush coleslaw a frequent side dish on your menu. Cabbage is cheaper and more nutritious than iceberg lettuce.
- Don't buy precut vegetables. You'll be paying more for less, nutritionally speaking.

FRUITS
- Slice fresh fruit in season and then freeze it. You'll be all set to make your morning smoothies—without buying those expensive bags of frozen fruit!
- Buy fresh berries in season and freeze them to enjoy at a later date.

IT'S BEEN SAID . . .

I was in the bad habit of eating breakfast on the run—which meant buying a muffin and tall cup of coffee every day. I have saved money and my figure by making a switch. Now, I have a refreshing Fat Flush fruit smoothie for breakfast. Sometimes, I even make it the night before, freeze it, and grab it as I head out the door. By the time I get to work, my smoothie is the consistency of sorbet. Best of all, with the money I've saved, I've purchased some stylish, smaller clothes!

MINDY B., MINNESOTA

HERBS AND SPICES

- Don't waste fresh herbs. Freeze them before they go bad and you have to throw them away.
- Some spices can be purchased in bulk for a lot less money. Be sure to check for the freshness of any bulk items before parting with your money.
- Don't toss out fresh ginger peels. Freeze them for later use in soups or broth.
- Experiment with all the Fat Flush herbs and spices. Seasonings help you economize by enhancing the taste of simple staple foods.

SURPRISING FAT FLUSH FOODS

- Almonds are in season in midsummer, so stock up on fresh bulk almonds at that time, seal them, and stick them in the freezer for year-round use.
- Buy plain yogurt (with live active cultures, of course) and flavor it yourself with your favorite Fat Flush fruits and seeds.

Above all, as you prepare your grocery list, keep in mind the connection between your health and the food you eat. In this regard, a simple old saying comes to mind: "You can pay now, or you can pay later." That fast-food burger off the dollar menu might seem like an inexpensive lunch, but it could cost you dearly in the long run. On the other hand, establishing eating habits that incorporate many or all of my 70 Fat Flush foods may help you avoid future medical expenses—and keep you slim, trim, and toned in the process.

Resources and Support

ONLINE SUPPORT

Please visit http://www.fatflush.com and http://www.annlouise.com for complete support on your Fat Flush journey and new lifestyle. Visitors to my website and subscribers to my e-mail list never miss my latest blogs and are the first to know about news and upcoming events. Plus you can stay up-to-date with my latest online webinars, articles, and radio and television appearances. Also, do join our Fat Flush community on Facebook at http://www.facebook.com/groups/fatflushcommunity/ for a 24/7 connection with other members, Fat Flush–friendly recipes, diet and exercise tips, testimonials, and motivation. The folks in this group are immeasurably generous in their support, advice, and knowledge!

UNI KEY HEALTH SYSTEMS

Uni Key Health Systems has been my go-to distributor for many supplements and test kits for over 25 years. It was founded in 1992 by James Templeton, a cancer survivor who used alternative medicine to heal himself and has since dedicated his life to helping others find the root causes of disease. Uni Key Health proudly provides high-quality, natural nutritional supplements, vitamins, and health information for diet and detox, weight loss, cleansing, antiaging, energy, hormonal balance, and skin care. I have been a spokesperson and formulator for Uni Key Health Systems for over 20 years.

181 West Commerce Drive
Hayden Lake, ID 83835
800.888.4353
http://www.unikeyhealth.com

Fat Flush–Compatible Supplements Available from Uni Key

- Bile Builder
- Carlson Fish Oil and Softgels
- CLA-1000
- Dandelion Root Tea
- Fat Flush Body Protein
- Fat Flush Whey Protein
- Flora-Key
- GLA-90
- Liver-Lovin Formula
- Mag-Key
- Melatonin 3 mg
- Omega Nutrition Cold Milled Flax Seeds
- Omega Nutrition Flaxseed Oil and Softgels
- ProgestaKey
- Super-GI Cleanse
- SweetLeaf Stevia
- Weight Loss Formula
- Whole Chia Seeds
- Y-C Cleanse

Also Available from Uni Key

- **Earthing products.** Reconnect to the earth's natural healing electrons with products designed to ground yourself for better sleep, increased endurance, enhanced energy, and overall balance.
- **Salivary hormone test.** Unlike blood tests, which do not measure bioavailable hormone activity, saliva testing is considered to be the most accurate measure of free, bioavailable hormonal activity. This personal hormone evaluation can be used to profile up to six hormones: estradiol, estriol, progesterone, testosterone, DHEA, and cortisol. Your personal results and a personal letter of recommendation from my office are mailed directly to your home.
- **Tissue mineral analysis.** This test uses a small sample of hair cut from the back of your head. The analysis includes a full report, up to 20 pages, which graphically shows the levels of 32 major minerals and 6 toxic metals in the body. Each mineral is fully evaluated in terms of its relationship with other minerals, which is a key to glandular function and metabolism rate. This report provides information on the effect of vitamin deficiency and excesses. There is also a complete discussion regarding environmental influences and disease tendencies based upon mineral levels and ratios. A list of recommended food

choices and supplements, based on the individual findings, is included at the end of the report.

- **Water filtration.** Purify your water to protect against harmful chemicals and toxins, parasites like giardia and amoeba, chloromines, and heavy metals. A free water quality consultation with a filtration expert is also available.

ADDITIONAL PRODUCTS

ASEA Global
6550 South Millrock Drive, Suite 100
Salt Lake City, UT 84121
http://www.aseaglobal.com

Over time, due to aging, stress, and environmental toxins, our bodies lose the ability to function at optimum levels. ASEA Redox Supplement is composed of the same life-sustaining molecules that exist in the human body, suspended in a pristine saline solution. It works at the cellular level to enhance function and assist your body's natural efforts to maximize energy and vitality.

Bibliography

GENERAL REFERENCES

Bowden, Jonny, *The 150 Healthiest Foods on Earth* (Beverly, MA: Fair Winds Press, 2017).

Boynton, Hilary, *The Heal Your Gut Cookbook* (White River Junction, VT: Chelsea Green Publishing, 2014).

Bragg, Paul C., and Patricia Bragg, *Apple Cider Vinegar* (Santa Barbara, CA: Health Science, 1995).

Burke, Valerie, "Is the Paleo Diet Right for You?," *Ancient Wisdom Meets Modern Science* (Amazon Digital Services, Kindle Edition, 2013).

Gittleman, Ann Louise, *The New Fat Flush Plan* (New York: McGraw-Hill, 2016).

Gittleman, Ann Louise, *The New Fat Flush Plan Cookbook* (New York: McGraw-Hill, 2017).

Reinhard, Tonia, *Superfoods: The Healthiest Foods on the Planet* (Richmond Hill, ON: Firefly Books, 2014).

Vanderhaeghe, Lorna R., *Healthy Fats for Life* (Kingston, ON: Quarry Health Books, 2003).

Ward, Bernard, *Healing Foods from the Bible* (Boca Raton, FL: American Media Mini Mags, 2001).

Williams, Anthony, *Medical Medium Life-Changing Foods* (Carlsbad, CA: Hay House, 2016).

Wood, Rebecca, *The New Whole Foods Encyclopedia* (New York: Penguin Books, 1999).

CHAPTER 1

Ali, N. M., et al., "The Promising Future of Chia, *Salvia hispanica* L.," *Journal of Biomedicine & Biotechnology* (November 21, 2012): 171956.

Al-Khalifa, A., et al., "Effect of Dietary Hempseed Intake on Cardiac Ischemia-Reperfusion Injury," *American Journal of Physiology* 292 (March 2007): R1198–R1203.

Ashton, O. B., et al., "Pigments in Avocado Tissue and Oil," *Journal of Agricultural and Food Chemistry* 54 (December 27, 2006): 10151–10158.

Assancao, M. L., et al., "Effects of Dietary Coconut Oil on the Biochemical and Anthropometric Profiles of Women Presenting Abdominal Obesity," *Lipids* 44 (July 2009): 593–601.

Ayerza, R., Jr., and W. Coates, "Effect of Dietary Alpha-Linolenic Fatty Acid Derived from Chia When Fed as Ground Seed, Whole Seed and Oil on Lipid Content and Fatty Acid Composition of Rat Plasma," *Annals of Nutrition & Metabolism* 51 (2007): 27–34.

Belleme, John, and Jan Belleme, *Culinary Treasures of Japan* (Garden City, NY: Avery Publishing Group Inc., 1992).

Buller, Amanda, Arizona State University, presented at the annual conference of American College of Nutrition in Orlando, FL, October 6, 2001.

Burger, O., et al., "Inhibition of *Helicobacter pylori* Adhesion to Human Gastric Mucus by a High-Molecular-Weight Constituent of Cranberry Juice," *Critical Reviews in Food Science & Nutrition* 42 (2002): 279–284.

Callaway J., et al., "Efficacy of Dietary Hempseed Oil in Patients with Atopic Dermatitis," *Journal of Dermatological Treatment* 16 (April 2005): 87–94.

Callaway, J. C., "Hempseed as a Nutritional Resource: An Overview," *Euphytica* 140 (January 2004): 65–72.

Carvajal-Zarrabal, O., et al., "Effect of Dietary Intake of Avocado Oil and Olive Oil on Biochemical Markers of Liver Function in Sucrose-Fed Rats," *BioMed Research International* (2014): 595479.

Cerino, V., "Chicken Soup for a Cold," Department of Public Relations, University of Nebraska Medical Center.

Chicco, A. G., et al., "Dietary Chia Seed (*Salvia hispanica* L.) Rich in Alpha-Linolenic Acid Improves Adiposity and Normalises Hypertriacylglycerolaemia and Insulin Resistance in Dyslipaemic Rats," *British Journal of Nutrition* 101 (January 2009): 41–50.

Clark, K. L., et al., "24-Week Study on the Use of Collagen Hydrolysate as a Dietary Supplement in Athletes with Activity-Related Joint Pain," *Current Medical Research and Opinion* 24 (May 2008): 1485–1496.

Dreher, M. L., and A. J. Davenport, "Hass Avocado Composition and Potential Health Effects," *Critical Reviews in Food Science and Nutrition* 53 (May 2013): 738–750.

Fernando, W. M., et al., "The Role of Dietary Coconut for the Prevention and Treatment of Alzheimer's Disease: Potential Mechanisms of Action." *British Journal of Nutrition* 114 (July 14, 2015): 1–14.

Girgih, A. T., et al., "Preventive and Treatment Effects of a Hemp Seed (*Cannabis sativa* L.) Meal Protein Hydrolysate Against High Blood Pressure in Spontaneously Hypertensive Rats," *European Journal of Nutrition* 53 (August 2014): 1237–1246.

Gittleman, Ann Louise, *The Fat Flush Plan* (New York: McGraw-Hill, 2002), 35.

Giuseppina, F., et al., "Gelatin Tannate Reduces the Proinflammatory Effects of Lipopolysaccharide in Human Intestinal Epithelial Cells," *Clinical and Experimental Gastroenterology* 5 (2012): 61–67.

Goodfriend, R., "Reduction of Bacteriuria and Pyuria Using Cranberry Juice," *Journal of the American Medical Association* 272 (August 1994): 589.

House, J. D., et al., "Evaluating the Quality of Protein from Hemp Seed (*Cannabis sativa* L.) Products Through the Use of the Protein Digestibility-Corrected Amino Acid Score Method," *Journal of Agricultural and Food Chemistry* 58 (November 24, 2010): 11801–11807.

Hu, Y., et al., "Coconut Oil: Non-Alternative Drug Treatment Against Alzheimer's Disease," *Nutrición Hospitalaria* 32 (December 1, 2015): 2822–2827.

Illian, T. G., et al., "Omega 3 Chia Seed Loading as a Means of Carbohydrate Loading," *Journal of Strength & Conditioning Research* 25 (January 2011): 61–65.

Li, X., et al., "A Meta-Analysis of the Efficacy and Safety of Using Oil Massage to Promote Infant Growth," *Journal of Pediatric Nursing* 31, no. 5 (September–October, 2016): e313–e322.

Liau, K. M., et al., "An Open-Label Pilot Study to Assess the Efficacy and Safety of Virgin Coconut Oil in Reducing Visceral Adiposity," *ISRN Pharmacology* 2011 (2011): 949686.

Lindeberg, S., and B. Lundh, "Apparent Absence of Stroke and Ischaemic Heart Disease in a Traditional Melanesian Island: A Clinical Study in Kitava," *Journal of Internal Medicine* 233 (March 1993): 269–275.

Lu, Q. Y., et al., "Inhibition of Prostate Cancer Cell Growth by an Avocado Extract: Role of Lipid-Soluble Bioactive Substances," *Journal of Nutritional Biochemistry* 16 (January 2005): 23–30.

Monro, J. A., et al., "The Risk of Lead Contamination in Bone Broth Diets," *Medical Hypotheses* 80 (April 2013): 389–390.

Oliveira, A. Paula de, et al., "Effect of Semisolid Formulation of *Persea americana* Mill (Avocado) Oil on Wound Healing in Rats," *Evidence-Based Complementary and Alternative Medicine*, 2013 (2013): 472382.

Padmanabhan, M., and G. Arumugam, "Effect of *Persea americana* (Avocado) Fruit Extract on the Level of Expression of Adiponectin and PPAR-γ in Rats Subjected to Experimental Hyperlipidemia and Obesity," *Journal of Complementary & Integrative Medicine* 11 (June 2014): 107–119.

Pedersen, C. B., et al., "Effects of Blueberry and Cranberry Juice Consumption on the Plasma Antioxidant Capacity of Healthy Female Volunteers," *European Journal of Clinical Nutrition* 54 (2000): 405–408.

Prior, I. A., et al., "Cholesterol, Coconuts, and Diet on Polynesian Atolls: A Natural Experiment: The Pukapuka and Tokelau Island Studies," *American Journal of Clinical Nutrition* 34 (August 1981): 1552–1561.

Prociuk, M. A., et al., "Cholesterol-Induced Stimulation of Platelet Aggregation Is Prevented by a Hempseed-Enriched Diet." *Canadian Journal of Physiology and Pharmacology* 86 (April 2008): 153–159.

Proksch, E., et al., "Oral Supplementation of Specific Collagen Peptides Has Beneficial Effects on Human Skin Physiology: A Double-Blind, Placebo-Controlled Study," *Skin Pharmacology and Physiology* 27 (2014): 47–55.

Rennard, B. O., et al., "Chicken Soup Inhibits Neutrophil Chemotaxis in Vitro," *Chest Journal* 118 (October 2000): 1150–1157.

Reyes-Caudillo, E., et al., "Dietary Fibre Content and Antioxidant Activity of Phenolic Compounds Present in Mexican Chia (*Salvia hispanica* L.) Seeds," *Food Chemistry* 107 (March 15, 2008): 656–663.

Rocha Filho, E. A., et al., "Essential Fatty Acids for Premenstrual Syndrome and Their Effect on Prolactin and Total Cholesterol Levels: A Randomized, Double Blind, Placebo-Controlled Study," *Reproductive Health* 8 (January 17, 2011).

Rosenblat, G., et al., "Polyhydroxylated Fatty Alcohols Derived from Avocado Suppress Inflammatory Response and Provide Non-Sunscreen Protection

Against UV-Induced Damage in Skin Cells," *Archives of Dermatological Research* 303 (May 2011): 239–246.

Sankaranarayanan, K., et al., "Oil Massage in Neonates: An Open Randomized Controlled Study of Coconut Versus Mineral Oil," *Indian Pediatrics* 42 (September 2005): 877–884.

Scaldaferri, F., et al., "Gelatin Tannate Ameliorates Acute Colitis in Mice by Reinforcing Mucus Layer and Modulating Gut Microbiota Composition: Emerging Role for 'Gut Barrier Protectors' in IBD?" *United European Gastroenterology Journal* 2 (April 2014): 113–122.

"Sprouting Chia Seeds," *The Happy Raw Kitchen*, May 24, 2010.

Stubbs R. J., and C. G. Harbron, "Covert, Manipulation of the Ratio of Medium- to Long-Chain Triglycerides in Isoenergetically Dense Diets: Effect on Food Intake in Ad Libitum Feeding Men," *International Journal of Obesity and Related Metabolic Disorders* 20 (May 1996): 435–444.

Stucker, M., et al., "Vitamin B(12) Cream Containing Avocado Oil in the Therapy of Plaque Psoriasis," *Dermatology* 203 (2001): 141–147.

Tennesen, M., "Drink to Your Health," *Health Magazine* 14 (June 2000): 88.

Unlu, N. Z., et al., "Carotenoid Absorption from Salad and Salsa by Humans Is Enhanced by the Addition of Avocado or Avocado Oil," *Journal of Nutrition* 135 (March 2005): 431–436.

Van Wymelbeke, V., et al., "Influence of Medium-Chain and Long-Chain Triacylglycerols on the Control of Food Intake in Men," *American Journal of Clinical Nutrition* 68 (August 1998): 226–234.

Vuksan, V., et al., "Reduction in Postprandial Glucose Excursion and Prolongation of Satiety: Possible Explanation of the Long-Term Effects of Whole Grain Salba (*Salvia hispanica* L.)," *European Journal of Clinical Nutrition* 64 (April 2010): 436–438.

Vuksan, V., et al., "Supplementation of Conventional Therapy with the Novel Grain Salba (*Salvia hispanica* L.) Improves Major and Emerging Cardiovascular Risk Factors in Type 2 Diabetes: Results of a Randomized Controlled Trial," *Diabetes Care* 30 (November 2007): 2804–2910.

Weiss, E. I., et al., "Inhibiting Interspecies Coaggregation of Plaque Bacteria with Cranberry Juice Constituent," *Journal of the American Dental Association* 129 (1998): 1719–1723.

Wien, M., et al., "A Randomized 3×3 Crossover Study to Evaluate the Effect of Hass Avocado Intake on Post-Ingestive Satiety, Glucose and Insulin Levels, and Subsequent Energy Intake in Overweight Adults," *Nutrition Journal* 12 (November 27, 2013): 155.

Yan, X., et al., "Characterization of Lignanamides from Hemp (*Cannabis sativa* L.) Seed and Their Antioxidant and Acetylcholinesterase Inhibitory Activities," *Journal of Agricultural and Food Chemistry* 63 (December 16, 2015): 10611–10619.

http://www.bottledwater.org.

CHAPTER 2

Bassano, L. A., et al., "Legume Consumption and Risk of Coronary Heart Disease in US Men and Women: NHANES I Epidemiologic Follow-Up Study," *Archives of Internal Medicine* 161 (November 2001): 2573–2578.

Geraedts, M. C., et al., "Validation of Using Chamber Technology to Study Satiety Hormone Release from Human Duodenal Specimens," *Obesity* 20 (March 2012): 678–682.

Gittleman, Ann Louise, *Eat Fat, Lose Weight* (Lincolnwood, IL: Keats Publishing, 1999), 60.

Kiatoko, M., et al., "Evaluating the Nutritional Status of Beef Cattle Herds from Four Soil Order Regions of Florida. I. Macroelements, Protein, Carotene, Vitamins A and E, Hemoglobin and Hematocrit," *Journal of Animal Science* 55 (July 1982): 28–37.

Jonsson, T., et al., "Agrarian Diet and Diseases of Affluence—Do Evolutionary Novel Dietary Lectins Cause Leptin Resistance?" *BMC Endocrine Disorders* 5 (2005): 1472–6825.

Joy, J. M., et al., "The Effects of 8 Weeks of Whey or Rice Protein Supplementation on Body Composition and Exercise Performance," *Nutrition Journal* 12 (June 20, 2013).

Kelemen, L. E., et al., "Associations of Dietary Protein with Disease and Mortality in a Prospective Study of Postmenopausal Women," *American Journal of Epidemiology* 161 (2005): 239–249.

Lanza, E., et al., "High Dry Bean Intake and Reduced Risk of Advanced Colorectal Adenoma Recurrence Among Participants in the Polyp Prevention Trial," *Journal of Nutrition* 136 (July 2006): 1896–1903.

Leaf, A., et al., "Clinical Prevention of Sudden Cardiac Death by N-3 Polyunsaturated Fatty Acids and Mechanism of Prevention of Arrhythmias by N-3 Fish Oils," *Circulation* 107 (June 2003): 2646–2652.

Li, S. S., et al., "Dietary Pulses, Satiety and Food Intake: A Systematic Review and Meta-Analysis of Acute Feeding Trials," *Obesity* 22 (August 2014): 1773–1789.

Orlich, M. J., et al., "Vegetarian Dietary Patterns and the Risk of Colorectal Cancers," *JAMA Internal Medicine* 175 (May 2015): 767–776.

Overduin, J., et al., "NUTRALYS® Pea Protein: Characterization of in Vitro Gastric Digestion and in Vivo Gastrointestinal Peptide Responses Relevant to Satiety," *Food & Nutrition Research* 59 (April 13, 2015): 25622.

Paddock, C., "Pea Protein Fights Blood Pressure and Kidney Disease," *Medical News Today*, March 23, 2009.

Villegas, R., et al., "Legume and Soy Food Intake and the Incidence of Type 2 Diabetes in the Shanghai Women's Health Study," *American Journal of Clinical Nutrition* 87 (January 2008): 162–167.

Wunjuntuk, K., et al., "Parboiled Germinated Brown Rice Protects Against CCl4-Induced Oxidative Stress and Liver Injury in Rats," *Journal of Medicinal Food* 19 (January 2016): 15–23.

Zhang, H., et al., "Lower Weight Gain and Hepatic Lipid Content in Hamsters Fed High Fat Diets Supplemented with White Rice Protein, Brown Rice Protein, Soy Protein, and Their Hydrolysates," *Journal of Agricultural and Food Chemistry* 59 (October 26, 2011): 10927–10933.

CHAPTER 3

Agarwal, S., et al., "Tomato Lycopene and Low-Density Lipoprotein Oxidation: A Human Dietary Intervention Study," *Lipids* 33 (1998): 981–984.

Anderson, Richard A., et al., "Elevated Intakes of Supplemental Chromium Improve Glucose and Insulin Variables in Individuals with Type 2 Diabetes," *Diabetes* 46 (November 1997): 1786.

Beet page, GreenMedInfo, http://www.greenmedinfo.com/substance/beet.

Cheney, Garnett, "Rapid Healing of Peptic Ulcers in Patients Receiving Fresh Cabbage Juice," *California Medicine* 70 (1949): 10.

Clifford, T., et al., "The Potential Benefits of Red Beetroot Supplementation in Health and Disease," *Nutrients* 7 (April 2015): 2801–2822.

Fahey, J. W., et al., "Sulforaphane Inhibits Extracellular, Intracellular, and Antibiotic-Resistant Strains of *Helicobacter pylori* and Prevents Benzopyrene-Induced Stomach Tumors," *Proceedings of the National Academy of Sciences* 99 (May 28, 2002): 7610–7615.

Ji, S., "Beet Juice Boosts Cognitive Function in One Dose," GreenMedInfo, June 30, 2015.

Krajka-Kuzniak, V., et al., "Beetroot Juice Protects Against N-Nitrosodiethylamine-Induced Liver Injury in Rats," *Food and Chemical Toxicology* 50, June 2012: 2027–2033.

Rimm, E. B., et al., "Folate and Vitamin B6 from Diet and Supplements in Relation to Risk of Coronary Heart Disease Among Women," *Journal of the American Medical Association* 279 (May 1998): 359–364.

Szaefer, H., et al., "Evaluation of the Effect of Beetroot Juice on DMBA-Induced Damage in Liver and Mammary Gland of Female Sprague-Dawley Rats," *Phytotherapy Research* 28 (January 2014): 55–61.

Velmurugan, S., et al., "Dietary Nitrate Improves Vascular Function in Patients with Hypercholesterolemia: A Randomized, Double-Blind, Placebo-Controlled Study." *American Journal of Clinical Nutrition* 103 (January 2016): 25–38. https://www.ncbi.nlm.nih.gov/pubmed/26607938.

CHAPTER 4

Ascherio, A., et al., "Intake of Potassium, Magnesium, Calcium, and Fiber and Risk of Stroke Among US Men," *Circulation* 98 (September 22, 1998): 1198–1204.

Asgary, S., et al., "Clinical Evaluation of Blood Pressure Lowering, Endothelial Function Improving, Hypolipidemic and Anti-Inflammatory Effects of Pomegranate Juice in Hypertensive Subjects," *Phytotherapy Research* 28 (February 2014): 193–199.

Asgary, S., et al., "Clinical Investigation of the Acute Effects of Pomegranate Juice on Blood Pressure and Endothelial Function in Hypertensive Individuals," *ARYA Atherosclerosis* 9 (November 2013): 326–331.

Bookheimer, S. Y., et al., "Pomegranate Juice Augments Memory and FMRI Activity in Middle-Aged and Older Adults with Mild Memory Complaints," *Evidence-Based Complementary and Alternative Medicine* (2013): 946298.

Colombo, E., et al., "A Review on the Anti-Inflammatory Activity of Pomegranate in the Gastrointestinal Tract," *Evidence-Based Complementary and Alternative Medicine* (2013): 247145.

Conrozier, T., et al., "A Complex of Three Natural Anti-Inflammatory Agents Provides Relief of Osteoarthritis Pain," *Alternative Therapies in Health and Medicine* 20 (Winter 2014): 32–37.

Dhandayuthapani, S., et al., "Bromelain-Induced Apoptosis in GI-101A Breast Cancer Cells," *Journal of Medicinal Food* 15 (April 2012): 344–349.

Fitzhugh, D. J., et al., "Bromelain Treatment Decreases Neutrophil Migration to Sites of Inflammation," *Clinical Immunology* 128 (July 2008): 66–74.

Gil, M. I., et al., "Antioxidant Activity of Pomegranate Juice and Its Relationship with Phenolic Composition and Processing," *Journal of Agricultural and Food Chemistry* 48 (October 2000): 4581–4589.

Glaser, D., and T. Hilberg, "The Influence of Bromelain on Platelet Count and Platelet Activity in Vitro," *Platelets* 17 (February 2006): 37–41.

Hartman, R. E., et al., "Pomegranate Juice Decreases Amyloid Load and Improves Behavior in a Mouse Model of Alzheimer's Disease," *Neurobiology of Disease* 24 (December 2006): 506–515.

Hosseini, B., et al., "Effects of Pomegranate Extract Supplementation on Inflammation in Overweight and Obese Individuals: A Randomized Controlled Clinical Trial," *Complementary Therapies in Clinical Practice* 22 (February 2016): 44–50.

Howarth, N. C., et al., "Dietary Fiber and Weight Regulation," *Nutrition Reviews* 59 (2001): 129–139.

Knekt, P., et al., "Flavonoid Intake and Coronary Mortality in Finland: A Cohort Study," *British Medical Journal* 312 (February 24, 1996): 478–481.

Le Marchand, L., et al., "Intake of Flavonoids and Lung Cancer," *Journal of the National Cancer Institute* 92 (2000): 154–160.

Mitsou, E. K., et al., "Effect of Banana Consumption on Faecal Microbiota: A Randomised, Controlled Trial," *Anaerobe* 17 (December 2011): 384–387.

Okoko, B. J., et al., "Childhood Asthma and Fruit Consumption," *European Respiratory Journal* 29 (2007): 1161–1168.

Pearson, D. A., et al., "Apple Juice Inhibits Low Density Lipoprotein Oxidation," *Life Sciences* 64 (1999): 1913–1920.

Pillai, K., et al., "Anticancer Effect of Bromelain with and Without Cisplatin or 5-FU on Malignant Peritoneal Mesothelioma Cells," *Anti-Cancer Drugs* 25 (February 2014): 50–160.

"Pomegranates: Three Steps No Mess Process," Pomegranate Council.

Rahnavelu, V., et al., "Potential Role of Bromelain in Clinical and Therapeutic Applications," *Biomedical Reports* 5 (September 2016): 283–288.

Rashidkhani, B., et al., "Fruits, Vegetables and Risk of Renal Cell Carcinoma: A Prospective Study of Swedish Women," *International Journal of Cancer* 113 (January 20, 2005): 451–455.

Sampath Kumar, K. P., et al., "Traditional and Medicinal Uses of Banana," *Journal of Pharmacognosy and Phytochemistry* 1 (2012): 51–63.

Secor, E. R., Jr., et al., "Bromelain Limits Airway Inflammation in an Ovalbumin-Induced Murine Model of Established Asthma," *Alternative Therapies in Health and Medicine* 18 (September–October 2012): 9–17.

Shukla, M., et al., "Bioavailable Constituents/Metabolites of Pomegranate (*Punica granatum* L) Preferentially Inhibit COX2 Activity ex Vivo and IL-1Beta-

Induced PGE2 Production in Human Chondrocytes in Vitro," *Journal of Inflammation* 5 (June 2008).

Tufts University, "Researching a Blueberry/Brain Power Connection," *Tufts University Health and Nutrition Letter* 19 (March 2001): 1.

Zarfeshany, A., et al., "Potent Health Effects of Pomegranate," *Advanced Biomedical Research* 3 (2014). https://www.ncbi.nlm.nih.gov/pmc/articles/PMC4007340/.

CHAPTER 5

Amsterdam, E., "My Dandelion Is a Flower," Elana's Pantry, 2016.

Berthold, H. K., et al., "Effect of a Garlic Oil Preparation on Serum Lipoproteins and Cholesterol Metabolism: A Randomized Controlled Trial," *Journal of the American Medical Association* 279 (1998): 1900–1902.

Broadhurst, C. L., et al., "Insulin-Like Biological Activity of Culinary and Medicinal Plant Aqueous Extracts in Vitro," *Journal of Agricultural Food Chemistry* 48 (March 2000): 849–852.

"Can Turmeric Prevent or Treat Cancer?" Cancer Research UK.

Chandran, B., and A. Goel, "A Randomized, Pilot Study to Assess the Efficacy and Safety of Curcumin in Patients with Active Rheumatoid Arthritis," *Phytotherapy Research* 26 (November 2012): 1719–1725.

Chatterjee, S. J., et al., "The Efficacy of Dandelion Root Extract in Inducing Apoptosis in Drug-Resistant Human Melanoma Cells," *Evidence-Based Complementary and Alternative Medicine* 2011 (2011): 129045.

Chithra, V., and S. Leelamma, "*Coriandrum sativum* Changes the Levels of Lipid Peroxides and Activity of Antioxidant Enzymes in Experimental Animals," *Indian Journal of Biochemistry and Biophysics* 36 (February 1999): 59–61.

Chithra, V., and S. Leelamma, "Hypolipidemic Effect of Coriander Seeds (*Coriandrum sativum*): Mechanism of Action," *Plant Foods for Human Nutrition* 51 (1997): 167–172.

Choi, U., et al., "Hypolipidemic and Antioxidant Effects of Dandelion (*Taraxacum officinale*) Root and Leaf on Cholesterol-Fed Rabbits," *International Journal of Molecular Science* 11 (2010): 67–78.

Clare, B. A., et al., "The Diuretic Effect in Human Subjects of an Extract of *Taraxacum officinale* Folium over a Single Day," *Journal of Alternative and Complementary Medicine* 15 (August 2009): 929–934.

Colquhoun, E., "Pungent Principles of Ginger (*Zingiber officinale*) Are Thermogenic in the Perfused Rat Hindlimb," *International Journal of Obesity* 16 (1992).

Dandelion page, GreenMedInfo.

Delaquis, P. J., et al., "Antimicrobial Activity of Individual and Mixed Fractions of Dill, Cilantro, Coriander and Eucalyptus Essential Oils," *International Journal of Food Microbiology* 74 (March 25, 2002): 101–109.

Fuhrman, B., et al., "Ginger Extract Consumption Reduces Plasma Cholesterol, Inhibits LDL Oxidation and Attenuates Development of Atherosclerosis in Atherosclerotic, Apolipoprotein E-Deficient Mice," *Journal of Nutrition* 130 (2000): 1124–1131.

Gonzalez-Castejon, M., et al., "Diverse Biological Activities of Dandelion," *Nutrition Reviews* 70 (September 2012): 534–547.

Kim, T., et al., "Curcumin Activates AMPK and Suppresses Gluconeogenic Gene Expression in Hepatoma Cells," *Biochemical and Biophysical Research Communications* 388 (October 16, 2009): 377–382.

Ostad, S. N., et al., "The Effect of Fennel Essential Oil on Uterine Contraction as a Model for Dysmenorrhea, Pharmacology, and Toxicology Study, *Journal of Ethnopharmacology* 76 (August 2001): 299–304.

Ovadje, P., et al., "Selective Induction of Apoptosis Through Activation of Caspase-8 in Human Leukemia Cells (Jurkat) by Dandelion Root Extract," *Journal of Ethnopharmacology* 133 (January 7, 2011): 86–91.

Pierro, D., et al., "Potential Role of Bioavailable Curcumin in Weight Loss and Omental Adipose Tissue Decrease: Preliminary Data of a Randomized, Controlled Trial in Overweight People with Metabolic Syndrome. Preliminary Study," *European Review for Medical and Pharmacological Sciences* 19 (November 2015): 4195–4202.

Portincasa, P., et al., "Curcumin and Fennel Essential Oil Improve Symptoms and Quality of Life in Patients with Irritable Bowel Syndrome," *Journal of Gastrointestinal and Liver Diseases* 25 (June 2016): 151–157.

Sahebkar, A., and Y. Henrotin, "Analgesic Efficacy and Safety of Curcuminoids in Clinical Practice: A Systematic Review and Meta-Analysis of Randomized Controlled Trials," *Pain Medicine* 17 (June 2016): 1192–1202.

Sanmukhani, J., et al., "Efficacy and Safety of Curcumin in Major Depressive Disorder: A Randomized Controlled Trial," *Phytotherapy Research* 28 (April 2014): 579–585.

Singh, G., et al., "Studies on Essential Oils: Part 10. Antibacterial Activity of Volatile Oils of Some Spices," *Phytotherapy Research* 7 (November 16, 2002): 680–682.

Taylor, R. A., and M. C. Leonard, "Curcumin for Inflammatory Bowel Disease: A Review of Human Studies," *Alternative Medicine Review* 16 (June 2011): 152–156.

"Turmeric Extract Suppresses Fat Tissue Growth in Rodent Models," *Tufts Now*, May 18, 2009.

Yoshioka, M., et al., "Effects of Red Pepper on Appetite and Energy Intake," *British Journal of Nutrition* 82 (1999): 115–123.

Zang, J., et al., "Pancreatic Lipase Inhibitory Activity of *Taraxacum officinale* in Vitro and in Vivo," *Nutrition Research and Practice* 2 (Winter 2008): 200–203.

Zhou, W., et al., "Clinical Research of Dandelion with Vancomycin Treating Methicillin-Resistant Coagulase-Negative Staphylococci Infection," *Journal of University of South China* (Medical Edition), issue 6 (2009).

http://www.sciencedaily.com/releases/1999/08/990806074926.htm.

CHAPTER 6

Abugoch, J. L. E., "Quinoa (*Chenopodium quinoa* Willd.): Composition, Chemistry, Nutritional, and Functional Properties," *Advances in Food and Nutrition Research* 58 (2009): 1–31.

Allouh, M. Z., et al., "Influence of *Cyperus esculentus* Tubers (Tiger Nut) on Male Rat Copulatory Behavior," *BMC Complementary Alternative Medicine* 15 (September 23, 2015): 331.

Arvill, A., and L. Bodin, "Effect of Short-Term Ingestion of Konjac Glucomannan on Serum Cholesterol in Healthy Men," *American Journal of Clinical Nutrition* 61 (March 1995): 585–589.

Azezli, A. D., et al., "The Use of Konjac Glucomannan to Lower Serum Thyroid Hormones in Hyperthyroidism," *Journal of the American College of Nutrition* 26 (December 2007): 663–668.

Badejo, A. A., et al., "Processing Effects on the Antioxidant Activities of Beverage Blends Developed from *Cyperus esculentus, Hibiscus sabdariffa,* and *Moringa oleifera* Extracts," *Preventative Nutrition Food Science* 19 (September 2014): 227–233.

Behall, K. M., et al., "Consumption of Both Resistant Starch and Beta-Glucan Improves Postprandial Plasma Glucose and Insulin in Women," *Diabetes Care* 29 (May 2006): 976–981.

Berti, C., et al., "In Vitro Starch Digestibility and in Vivo Glucose Response of Gluten-Free Foods and Their Gluten Counterparts," *European Journal of Nutrition* 43 (August 2004): 198–204.

Birt, D. F., et al., "Resistant Starch: Promise for Improving Human Health," *Advances in Nutrition* 4 (November 2013): 587–601.

Ekeanyanwu, R. C., and C. I. Ononogbu, "Nutritive Value of Nigerian Tigernut (*Cyperus esculentus* L.)," *Agricultural Journal* 5 (2010): 297–302.

Fortes, C., et al., "Diet and Overall Survival in a Cohort of Very Elderly People," *Epidemiology* 11 (July 2000): 440–445.

Fraser, G. E., "Nut Consumption, Lipids, and Risk of a Coronary Event," *Clinical Cardiology* 22, suppl. S3 (July 1999): 11–5.

Gargari, B. P., et al., "Is There Any Place for Resistant Starch, as Alimentary Prebiotic, for Patients with Type 2 Diabetes?" *Complementary Therapies in Medicine* 23 (December 2015): 810–815.

Genta, S., et al., "Yacon Syrup: Beneficial Effects on Obesity and Insulin Resistance in Humans," *Clinical Nutrition* 28 (April 2009): 182–187.

Gentile, C. L., et al., "Resistant Starch and Protein Intake Enhances Fat Oxidation and Feelings of Fullness in Lean and Overweight/Obese Women," *Nutrition Journal* 14 (October 29, 2015).

"Growing Andean Root Crops: Yacón," University of California Master Gardeners of San Mateo and San Francisco. http://smsf-mastergardeners.ucanr.edu/Elkus/Growing_Yacón/.

"I've Fallen for Tigernuts (and a Recipe for Nigerian-Style Tigernut Milk)," Nourished Kitchen. http://nourishedkitchen.com/tigernut-milk-kunnu-aya/.

Johnston, K. L., et al., "Resistant Starch Improves Insulin Sensitivity in Metabolic Syndrome," *Diabetic Medicine* 27 (April 2010): 391–397.

Kendall, Z., "Yacon Syrup," Permaculture Research Institute, August 16, 2011.

Lobo, A. R., et al., "Effects of Fructans-Containing Yacon (*Smallanthus sonchifolius* Poepp and Endl.) Flour on Caecum Mucosal Morphometry, Calcium and Magnesium Balance, and Bone Calcium Retention in Growing Rats," *British Journal of Nutrition* 97 (April 2007): 776–785.

Loening-Baucke, V., et al., "Fiber (Glucomannan) Is Beneficial in the Treatment of Childhood Constipation," *Pediatrics* 113 (March 2004): e259–264.

Macho, G. A., "Baboon Feeding Ecology Informs the Dietary Niche of *Paranthropus boisei*," *PLOS ONE* 9 (January 8, 2014).

Pasko, P., et al., "Effect of Quinoa Seeds (*Chenopodium quinoa*) in Diet on Some Biochemical Parameters and Essential Elements in Blood of High Fructose-Fed Rats," *Plant Foods for Human Nutrition* 65 (December 2010): 333–338.

Peng, S. S., et al., "Long-Term Animal Feeding Trial of the Refined Konjac Meal. II. Effects of the Refined Konjac Meal on the Aging of the Brain, Liver, and Cardiovascular Tissue Cells in Rats," *Biomedical and Environmental Sciences* 8 (March 1995): 80–87.

Ranilla, L. G., et al., "Evaluation of Indigenous Grains from the Peruvian Andean Region for Antidiabetes and Antihypertension Potential Using in Vitro Methods," *Journal of Medicinal Food* 12 (August 2009): 704–713.

Ruales, J., and B. M. Nair, "Nutritional Quality of the Protein in Quinoa (*Chenopodium quinoa*, Willd) Seeds," *Plant Foods for Human Nutrition* 42 (January 1992): 1–11.

Sanchez-Zapata, E., et al., "Tiger Nut (*Cyperus esculentus*) Commercialization: Health Aspects, Composition, Properties, and Food Applications," *Comprehensive Reviews in Food Science and Food Safety* 11 (July 2012): 366–377.

Sood, N., et al., "Effect of Glucomannan on Plasma Lipid and Glucose Concentrations, Body Weight, and Blood Pressure: Systematic Review and Meta-Analysis," *American Journal of Clinical Nutrition* 88 (October 2008): 1167–1175.

Valentova, K., et al., "The Effect of *Smallanthus sonchifolius* Leaf Extracts on Rat Hepatic Metabolism," *Cell Biology and Toxicology* 20 (March 2004): 109–120.

Valentova, K., et al., "Induction of Glucokinase mRNA by Dietary Phenolic Compounds in Rat Liver Cells in Vitro," *Journal of Agricultural and Food Chemistry* 55 (September 19, 2007): 7726–7731.

Vega-Galvez, A., et al., "Nutrition Facts and Functional Potential of Quinoa (*Chenopodium quinoa* Willd.), an Ancient Andean Grain: A Review," *Journal of Science and Food and Agriculture* 90 (December 2010): 2541–1547.

Wien, M., "Almonds vs. Complex Carbohydrates in a Weight Reduction Program," *International Journal of Obesity* 27 (November 2003): 1356–1372.

Wu, W. T., et al., "Ameliorative Effects of Konjac Glucomannan on Human Faecal β-Glucuronidase Activity, Secondary Bile Acid Levels and Faecal Water Toxicity Towards Caco-2 Cells," *British Journal of Nutrition* 105 (February 2011): 593–600.

Zemel, M. B., et al., "Dairy (Yogurt) Augments Fat Loss and Reduces Central Adiposity During Energy Restriction in Obese Subjects," *Federation of American Societies for Experimental Biology* 17 (2003): A1088.

CHAPTER 7

"A New (Painful) World Record? Woman Has 12,000 Gallstones Removed in Surgery," *Huffington Post*, November 30, 2015.

Aabdallah, D. M., and N. I. Eid, "Possible Neuroprotective Effects of Lecithin and Alpha-Tocopherol Alone or in Combination Against Ischemia/Reperfusion

Insult in Rat Brain," *Journal of Biochemical and Molecular Toxicology* 18 (2004): 273–278.

Adams, J. B., et al., "Nutritional and Metabolic Status of Children with Autism vs. Neurotypical Children, and the Association with Autism Severity," *Nutrition & Metabolism* 8 (June 8, 2011): 34.

ASEA Product Usage Guide, ASEA, 2013.

Bahadoran, Z., et al., "Effect of Broccoli Sprouts on Insulin Resistance in Type 2 Diabetic Patients: A Randomized Double-Blind Clinical Trial," *International Journal of Food Sciences and Nutrition* 63 (November 2012): 767–771.

Blankson, H., et al., "Conjugated Linoleic Acid Reduces Body Fat Mass in Overweight and Obese Human," *Journal of Nutrition* 130, issue 12 (2000): 2943–2948.

Chiu, H. Y., et al., "Effects of Intravenous and Oral Magnesium on Reducing Migraine: A Meta-Analysis of Randomized Controlled Trials," *Pain Physician* 19 (January 2014): E97–112.

Collins, Y., et al., "Mitochondrial Redox Signalling at a Glance," *Journal of Cell Science* 125 (2012): 801–806.

"Contamination a Common Problem in 'Greens' and 'Whole Foods' Products According to ConsumerLab.com," ConsumerLab Press Release, July 8, 2013.

Dibaba, D. T., et al., "Dietary Magnesium Intake and Risk of Metabolic Syndrome: A Meta-Analysis," *Diabetes Medicine* 31 (November 2014): 1301–1309.

Filippin, L. I., et al., "Redox Signalling and the Inflammatory Response in Rheumatoid Arthritis," *Clinical & Experimental Immunology* 152 (June 2008): 415–422.

Funfstuck, R., et al., "Prevent Reinfection by L-Methionine in Patients with Recurrent Urinary Tract Infection," *Medizinische Klinik* 92 (1997): 574–581.

Goden, G., et al., "Excessive Caloric Intake Acutely Causes Oxidative Stress, GLUT4 Carbonylation, and Insulin Resistance in Healthy Men," *Science Translational Medicine* 7, September 9, 2015.

Gruy-Kapral, C., et al., "Conjugated Bile Acid Replacement Therapy for Short-Bowel Syndrome," *Gastroenterology* 116 (January 1999): 15–21.

Guerrerio, A. L., et al., "Choline Intake in a Large Cohort of Patients with Nonalcoholic Fatty Liver Disease," *American Journal of Clinical Nutrition* 95 (April 2012): 892–900.

Hellhammer, J., et al., "Effects of Soy Lecithin Phosphatidic Acid and Phosphatidylserine Complex (PAS) on the Endocrine and Psychological Responses to Mental Stress," *Stress* 7 (June 2004): 119–126.

Hofve, J., "Redox Signaling: The Anti-Aging Breakthrough," *Little Big Cat*, August 31, 2011.

Hruby, A., et al., "Higher Magnesium Intake Is Associated with Lower Fasting Glucose and Insulin, with No Evidence of Interaction with Select Genetic Loci, in a Meta-Analysis of 15 CHARGE Consortium Studies," *Journal of Nutrition* 143 (March 2013): 345–353.

Hsu, C. L., and G. C. Yen, "Effects of Flavonoids and Phenolic Acids on the Inhibition of Adipogenesis in 3T3-L1 Adipocytes," *Journal of Agricultural and Food Chemistry* 55 (September 2007): 8404–8410.

Ji, S., "Magnesium's Importance Far Greater Than Previously Imagined," GreenMedInfo.com, December 5, 2012.

Kaats, G., et al., "A Randomized, Double-Masked, Placebo-Controlled Study of the Effects of Chromium Picolinate Supplementation on Body Composition: A Replication and Extension of a Previous Study," *Current Therapeutic Research* 59(1998): 379–388.

Laidlaw, S. A., et al., "Plasma and Urine Taurine Levels in Vegans," *American Journal of Clinical Nutrition* 47 (April 1988): 660–663.

Mazur, A., et al., "Magnesium and the Inflammatory Response: Potential Physiopathological Implications," *Archives of Biochemistry and Biophysics* 458 (February 1, 2007): 48–56.

Mercola, J., "Choline: Why You Should Eat Your Egg Yolks and Take Krill," Mercola.com, July 18, 2106.

Miranda, D. T., et al., "Soy Lecithin Supplementation Alters Macrophage Phagocytosis and Lymphocyte Response to Concanavalin A: A Study in Alloxan-Induced Diabetic Rats," *Cell Biochemistry and Function* 26 (December 2008): 859–865.

Moghadam, M. H., et al., "Antihypertensive Effect of Celery Seed on Rat Blood Pressure in Chronic Administration," *Journal of Medicinal Food* 16 (June 2013): 558–563.

Mourad, A. M., et al., "Influence of Soy Lecithin Administration on Hypercholesterolemia," *Cholesterol* 2010 (2010): 824813.

Otsuki, T., et al., "Changes in Arterial Stiffness and Nitric Oxide Production with Chlorella-Derived Multicomponent Supplementation in Middle-Aged and Older Individuals," *Journal of Clinical Biochemistry and Nutrition* 57 (November 2015): 228–232.

Pariza, M. W., "Conjugated Linoleic Acid May Be Useful in Treating Diabetes by Controlling Body Fat and Weight Gain," *Diabetes Technology and Therapy* 4 (2002): 335–338.

Qu, X., et al., "Magnesium and the Risk of Cardiovascular Events: A Meta-Analysis of Prospective Cohort Studies," *PLOS ONE* 8 (March 8, 2013).

Ripps, H., and W. Shen, "Review: Taurine: A 'Very Essential' Amino Acid," *Molecular Vision* 18 (2012): 2673–2686.

Schwartz, R., et al., "Magnesium Absorption in Human Subjects from Leafy Vegetables, Intrinsically Labeled with Stable 26Mg," *American Journal of Clinical Nutrition* 39 (April 1984): 571–576.

"Scientists Close in on Taurine's Activity in the Brain," *Medical News Today*, January 18, 2008.

Sircus, M., "Inflammation and Pain Management with Magnesium," DrSircus.com, December 8, 2009.

Sircus, M., "Magnesium Warnings and Contraindications," DrSircus.com, February 10, 2011.

Takihara, K., et al., "Beneficial Effect of Taurine in Rabbits with Chronic Congestive Heart Failure," *American Heart Journal* 112 (December 1986): 1278–1284.

Toouli, J., et al., "Gallstone Dissolution in Man Using Cholic Acid and Lecithin," *Lancet* 2 (December 6, 1975): 1124–1126.

Tsuboyama-Kasaoka, N., et al., "Taurine (2-Aminoethanesulfonic Acid) Deficiency Creates a Vicious Circle Promoting Obesity," *Endocrinology* 147 (July 2006): 3276–3284.

Wang, D. Q. H., and M. C. Carey, "Therapeutic Uses of Animal Biles in Traditional Chinese Medicine: An Ethnopharmacological, Biophysical Chemical and Medicinal Review," *World Journal of Gastroenterology* 20 (August 7, 2014): 9952–9975.

Wark, P., et al., "Magnesium Intake and Colorectal Tumor Risk: A Case-Control Study and Meta-Analysis," *American Journal of Clinical Nutrition* 96 (September 2012): 622–631.

Zhang, M., et al., "Beneficial Effects of Taurine on Serum Lipids in Overweight or Obese Non-Diabetic Subjects," *Amino Acids* 26 (June 2004): 267–271.

Index

About the Author

Ann Louise Gittleman, PhD, CNS, is undisputedly the First Lady of Nutrition. As a nutritional visionary and health pioneer, she has fearlessly stood on the front lines of diet and detox, the environment, and women's health. *Self* magazine describes her as one of the Top Ten Notable Nutritionists in the United States, and thousands of nutritionists, health coaches, and practitioners have benefited from her work.

Years before the Paleo, ketogenic, and vegan diet trends, in her first book, *Beyond Pritikin* (1988), Ann Louise was the very first to proclaim that obesity and diabetes were caused by a lack of the right type of fat and an excess of the wrong kind of carbohydrates, including gluten-rich grain. She was also the first nutritionist to write about the perils of gluten and discuss the blood-type theory in 1996, boldly stating, in her book *Your Body Knows Best*, that one diet may not be right for everyone.

She has also been a tireless crusader for women by offering natural solutions to menopause and perimenopausal symptoms, decades before anybody else, in her award-winning *Super Nutrition for Women*, as well as *Super Nutrition for Menopause* and her *New York Times* bestseller *Before the Change*.

She then revolutionized dieting in the first edition of *The Fat Flush Plan*—an international bestseller—by proclaiming that the liver was the body's primary fat-burning organ (and detoxifier).

Most recently, she led the charge against the hidden hazards of cell phones, iPads, smart meters, and WiFi in her groundbreaking book *Zapped*.

She has appeared on *20/20*, *Dr. Phil*, *The View*, *Good Morning America*, *Extra!*, *FitTV*, and *The Early Show*. In addition, her work has been featured on ABC, CNN, PBS, CBS, NBC, MSNBC, CBN, Fox News, and the BBC.

She has served as a celebrity spokesperson and formula developer for many of the leading companies in the health foods and network marketing industry. Her work has been featured in a myriad of national publications including *Time*, *Newsweek*, *Glamour*, and the *New York Times*.

ENGAGING HEALTH

Today she continues to dedicate herself to carving out new landmarks in functional and integrative medicine with her latest e-book, *Eat Fat, Lose*

Weight. She is a popular speaker on Internet summits and is actively involved with videos and her blog. Her expert advice often appears in *First for Women* magazine, where she was the nutrition columnist for more than 10 years.

In 2016 Ann Louise was presented with the Humanitarian Award from the Cancer Control Society. She currently sits on the Advisory Board for the International Institute for Building-Biology & Ecology, the Nutritional Therapy Association, Inc., and Clear Passage, Inc.

Connect with Ann Louise at www.annlouise.com, www.fatflush.com, and facebook.com/annlouisegittleman.

Books from Award-Winning Pioneer Nutritionalist Ann Louise Gittleman, PH.D, C.N.S.

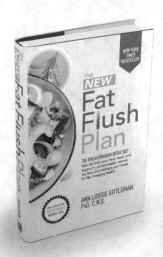

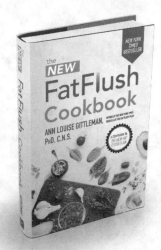

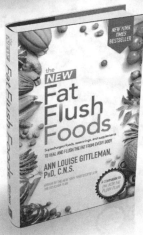

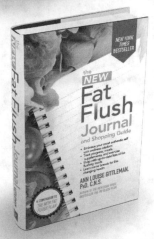